FRONTOTEMPORAL RELATED DEMENTIAS

Behavioral Variant
Frontotemporal Dementia
(bvFTD) & Progressive
Supranuclear Palsy (PSP)

JERRY BELLER HEALTH RESEARCH
INSTITUTE

DEDICATION

To people living with Dementia and their loved ones.

CONTENTS

ACKNOWLEDGMENTS

Thanks to the American Academy of Neurology, Atlanta Center for Medical Research, Alzheimer's Association, Alzheimer's Disease Center, Alzheimer's Disease Center of Northwestern University, Alzheimer's Foundation of America, American Academy of Neurology, Association for Frontotemporal Degeneration, Australia Neurological Research, CDC, Department of Health and Human Services, Duke University Medical Center, Emory Hospital, Harvard Medical School, Johns Hopkins Medicine, Mayo Clinic, National Aphasia Association, National Institute of Neurological Disorders and Strokes, National Library of Medicine, National Institute on Aging, National Institutes of Health, Prince of Wales Medical Research Institute, *PubMed*, Stanford Library School of Medicine, Stanford Medicine, UCSF Department of Neurology, UCSF Memory and Aging Center, University of Cambridge Neurology Unit, World Health Organization (WHO), *Journal of American Medical Association* (JAMA), and several other organizations that provided information used for this book. Thanks to everybody who assisted this book in a variety of important ways, and everybody at Beller Health Research Institute. To my editor, John Briggs, who helps me improve every book. To all sources and for the photos. Most of all, thanks to my wife, Nicola Beller

FOREWORD

Before diving into the book's subject matter, let's discuss two related Dementia series:

- *2020 Dementia Overview* series
- *2020 Dementia Types, Symptoms, Stages, & Risk Factors* series

2020 Dementia Overview series is an extension of the medical groundbreaking *19 Dementia Types, Symptoms, Stages, & Risk Factors* series, the first covering all primary dementia types.

After spending decades building an audience in other genres, including nutrition, circumstances turned the world upside down. Doctors diagnosed my mother with Alzheimer's. The same doctors soon diagnosed my father with cancer. A few months later, my father's favorite brother and my closest uncle died.

Three consecutive hard blows blew the world beyond recognition.

Tough and decent as they come, dad insisted on taking care of my mother while fighting brain cancer. My brothers and sister-in-law did their share, but Dad cared for my mother for a long time while they worked. Dad proved what a remarkable and great man he was down the stretch but finally succumbed to brain cancer.

My brothers and sister-in-law did their best to take care of mom, but it came at a price. Caregiving for a dementia patient is an indescribable horror I would not wish on my worst enemy.

You must watch somebody you love wilt away, little by little until dementia wipes away huge chunks of their personality.

Living away, my wife and I visited when possible. We saw how mom deteriorated, but also the effect caregiving had on my father and brothers. It was like watching a train wreck over and over, each time getting worse and helpless to prevent it.

Watching Alzheimer's takedown, my strong-willed mother and others bruised my soul. My writing shifted initially to learn about Alzheimer's, but the more learned, the more I cringed.

The cold hard facts rendered me speechless. Over 5.8 million Americans, and 44 million people worldwide, suffer Alzheimer's. No cure. Just a devastating and expensive slow march towards an agonizing end.

Not content to kill, Alzheimer's tortured Mom for years before killing her. It robbed her memory and damaged her brain, where she repeated herself in a continuous loop, each time thinking she was saying it the first time. As the disease advanced, the neurological disorder destroyed her mind and body.

Seeing dementia take down that tough old bird rattled me. While I could not bring back my mother, I dedicate my life to researching and writing about dementia 8-12 hours per day, six or seven days per week.

I tackled Alzheimer's to learn everything I could about the brute and determine how I and others might prevent it and other noncommunicable diseases. Having written on nutrition and advocated health in Washington, I already had a clue but determined to figure out how to prevent Alzheimer's. But I needed to know more, much more, about this terrorizing neurological disorder.

I learned Alzheimer's was just one of over one-hundred neurological disorders causing dementia. When I searched for a book covering the primary dementias, none existed. Instead, I turned to individual books and again found no books written on several of the most frequent dementias.

In what on the one hand seems like yesterday and the other a lifetime ago, I set out several years ago to write a dementia book covering the 15 most prevalent dementia types. The first to do that, I next wrote books covering each of the 15 most prevalent dementias.

In 2020, I expanded the book covering 15 dementias to 19 dementia types. I also released books on each of the 19 dementias. While proud of these medical firsts, I do not take myself too seriously.

As one of the dozens of scientists, neurologists, researchers, and writers who devote their lives to fighting the war against dementia, I remain humble. I appreciate the individual and combined accomplishments of everybody else in the field.

Nor should any of us get cocky knowing we're losing the war. If we win the war during my lifetime, I will celebrate with hundreds of people worldwide who helped defeat the great beast of our day.

My two-book series break medical ground, and I consider major achievements but remain two among hundreds of significant contributions to the dementia field by people around the globe.

The series provides patients and loved ones a great resource for dementias not covered as extensive as Alzheimer's and the more prevalent types.

By covering the 19 most prevalent dementias, doctors, nurses, and medical professionals benefit from a series covering neurological disorders causing 99% of dementia. The series helps primary care physicians, providers, and nurses who struggle to diagnose dementias with overlapping symptoms.

The series is an organic, evolving work, and each book receives major annual updates. As science uncovers information, we add important data in new editions. We also polish each edition.

We describe the writing goal in three ways:
1. Simplify the language and make it easier for nonscientists to comprehend.
2. Honor the science and facts.
3. Document science and include citations for doctors,

nurses, medical researchers, students, and patients.

Our goal is to provide invaluable medical information for professionals, patients, loved ones, and caregivers.

I do not reinvent the wheel but accumulate the best research and teach our readers a better understanding of Alzheimer's and the other 18 primary dementia types.

Among the worst news is one of our loved ones has dementia. A killer disease with no cure frightens the bravest souls.

This medical condition destroys, not just the inflicted, but their loved ones. Besides the patient, nobody suffers more than voluntary caregivers. Watching a mother, father, brother, sister, wife, or husband suffering dementia brutalizes the soul.

I study dementia year around to write and release annual updates to honor people—including my mother—taken by Alzheimer's or one of the other primary dementias.

Modest book royalties are the only compensation, as I accept no money from corporations to promote their product. Nor do I have an ax to grind with anybody in the medical profession.

Having written 100 plus books over four decades, I am thankful to readers for collectively providing me a decent income. However, now in my sixties, I care little about riches and fame.

Who is the reading audience?

The audience falls into five categories.

Those Diagnosed with Dementia

If doctors diagnose you with dementia, my heart goes out to you. You're in for a long battle. Do yourself a favor and focus on slowing the disease and extending the quality of life. One word of caution, the books in this series speak to not only patients, but also families, doctors, students, nurses, and caregivers. Many of those diagnosed with dementia appreciate and benefit from the books, but some find some of the material too disturbing. I intend to write books exclusively for patients but must finish the work related to this series first. While there is not anything too shocking, I wrote the material for a wide audience, meaning I am not always speaking to patients specifically. I promise to personalize an edition for patients and loved ones after finishing this series. By shining a light on all 19 primary dementia types, I hope to help the medical community better distinguish and diagnose neurological disorders.

Loved Ones of Those Diagnosed

If doctors diagnose a loved one with dementia, he or she needs you more than ever. Depending on the type, dementia causes behavioral problems, memory issues, motor decline, and other psychological and physical disorders. The learning curve is steep and changes as one moves from one stage to the next. As with those with dementia, I warn families these books provide a technical overview, and the emphasis is not always on the emotional aspect. If you want to learn about dementias, this series is a great option. If you're looking more for emotional support, there are more appropriate books. I also plan to write a book specifically for families once fulfilling responsibilities for this series.

Medical Professionals

If you are a medical professional interested in studying the dementias, the series covers the dementias responsible for 99% of dementia. While neurologists probably already know the 19 primary dementias, the books provide a quick overview and reference for primary care physicians, nurses, other medical professionals, and students. I also include citations so you can continue your investigation beyond the book's scope.

Volunteer & Professional Caregivers

If you are a dementia caregiver, you are also in for a long, difficult march. Dementia patients demand 24/7 care in later stages, requiring help to go to the bathroom, bathing, and other basic daily functions. While this series is not written solely for caregiving, caregivers benefit by gaining a better understanding of each dementia, their symptoms, and progression.

Anybody Wanting to Learn About A Disease That Strikes 1 Of 6 Americans, And 1 Of 3 Seniors

The series benefits anybody who wants to gain an intermediate understanding of the 19 dementias.

Series' First Lesson

Doctors, like teachers, are part of a sacred profession. **Nothing I say or write replaces your need for a competent doctor!** Nor does any criticism of the profession diminish my respect and admiration for the best.

I detest the worst teachers who fail students and society but love and respect the best. Society would crumble without the most devoted and competent teachers.

Similar, I abhor incompetent, greedy doctors who fail patients and society, but love and respect the best.

The profession must weed out incompetent, uncaring, corrupt doctors, and medical personnel. Every profession has a percentage of bad apples, but within the medical profession, they are cancerous!

Nothing good I write about the medical profession includes incompetent, uncaring doctors, researchers, nurses, etc. And nothing bad I write targets the best.

The series criticizes the profession when deserved, but the first lesson in this series: **Find a competent doctor!** If you have one, count your blessings. If not, find one.

Just as one can learn outside the classroom, we live in a blessed age where medical information is available for anybody on the internet. Such information serves us well, but do not—for a minute-think it replaces the need for a competent, devoted doctor.

The Wrong Doctors

Let me begin this section by saying I love and respect quality doctors, nurses, researchers, and medical professionals from the bottom of my heart and the fullness of my mind.

However, this section is not about what's right in the medical profession.

Glorified idiots, bad doctors are dangerous parasites who dishonor a noble profession. Smart enough to finish medical school, but greedy or flawed beyond redemption, they are like priests working for the devil. Among the worse members of society are doctors motivated by greed or limited by incompetence. Walking parasites!

The Wrong Doctors + Big Pharm + Big Insurance + Big Hospital = Expensive & Inadequate Health Care

Over the past few decades, Big pharmaceuticals, Big Insurance, and their political puppets appointed doctors sanctioned drug dealers. Entrusting the worse doctors with such powers produces little or no better results than assigning the task to a thug on the worst corner in America.

The worst doctors who hand out drugs like candy serve nobody's purpose but their own and Big Pharm.

Not an indictment of the entire profession, but unfortunately, Big Insurance dictates the typical office visit includes a quick examination and one or more prescriptions. The approach is not based on good science and runs counter to everything science teaches us.

What About Some Tough Love?

The one thing people today do not want is what we often need most, tough love. People want everything sugarcoated and easy.

The problem is most of the time; life is neither sweet nor easy.

What patients need much of the time is not an alleged "magic pill," but instead tough love. Doctors must learn nutrition and teach patients to eat healthier, exercise more, and get 7-8 hours of sleep per night. Like it or not, this is part of modern medicine. Showing up and passing out pills all day is not preventing Alzheimer's and other dementias, nor curing them.

Medical professionals must lead by example and embrace the science of nutrition, exercise, and sleep. If a healthy diet and exercise are the two cornerstones to health, the third is sleep.

The average person needs few or no drugs if they practice healthy habits.

Any doctor who does not vigorously advocate a balanced whole food diet, exercise most days of the week, and 7-8 hours' sleep per night neglects their duty and

Instead, too many doctors ignore the three cornerstones of health and are content to write their patients unnecessary and potentially dangerous prescriptions for the rest of their lives. 100% emphasis on treating symptoms with drugs, which often require more drugs to counter the side effects, is producing disastrous results. To be the best doctor, one must also emphasize prevention.

Failed Drug Trials

None of the drug trials have produced even one drug that cures Alzheimer's and other dementias. While science has failed to produce any effective dementia drugs, scientific studies prove we can do much by practicing healthy habits to slow or reduce our dementia risk.

The Medical Profession Must Think Outside the Box

The hopeless circle of failed drug trials demands we think outside the box or, as neurologist David Perlmutter advocates, expand the box. He and other neurologists deserve credit for recognizing medicine is failing the dementia war and rocking the boat of conventional wisdom. I must not agree with every point "maverick" neurologists like David Perlmutter, Dale Bredesen, and Deepak Chopra make to respect them for turning conventional wisdom on its head.

Conventional wisdom is losing the Alzheimer's and dementia war!

Not Anti-doctors or Anti-drugs

I am not anti-doctors or anti-drugs and do not understand those who insist neither are needed. I revere competent doctors who practice and advocate the three cornerstones of health. I also recognize the polio vaccine and many other drugs as nothing short of miraculous.

But, my love for what is right about the medical profession will not silence me about what is wrong. And, pretending drugs are the answer to defeating Alzheimer's or dementia is a colossal failure.

You cannot "**do no harm**" and write prescription drugs at the volume of the average doctor.

Choose A Doctor with The Same Care as You Do A Spouse

Find a competent, dedicated, caring, experienced, informed, ethical doctor who listens and respects your opinion, and writes prescriptions as a LAST RESORT.

Without the right doctor, you are at the mercy of a profit-oriented health system that seldom puts the patient's interests first, second, or third.

Nothing I say or write in these books or elsewhere means you should not see a doctor, stop taking your medication, or otherwise undermine the medical profession's ability to diagnose and treat any medical symptoms you might experience.

Find a good doctor you trust with your life and ask him or her pointed questions concerning your health and any treatment they recommend.

Outside the Bubble

I challenge the medical profession where necessary, just as I criticize Congress and the United States government for their mistakes or shortcomings. My brief career as a Congressional staffer taught me how difficult it is to maintain one's focus inside the bubble.

Seeing the big picture is no less challenging inside the medical bubble motivated by profit.

Profiteers fund too many studies to promote their product or discredit somebody else's. Blatant self-interests taint studies and confuse the public. Such contradictory studies confuse and make it impossible for the average person to understand which studies to believe.

I respect ethical, competent, dedicated, and hardworking nurses, doctors, and other medical personnel. As much as I criticize what is wrong within the profession, I cannot praise the majority of medical professionals often enough. Getting quality medical care when we need it is one of life's greatest blessings.

Nor do I object to medical-related businesses making a reasonable profit in return for needed medical supplies and services.

Nor should any competent and ethical medical professionals object to anybody challenging medical incompetence and profiteers.

Trust Thy Doctor

The right doctor does not discriminate between physical and mental diseases, so hold back nothing if you or a loved one exhibits symptoms.

If you lack the right doctor, find the right one. Outside you and the daily habits you establish, nobody is more important than your doctor for your health. You must be able to tell him or her medical information you might be reluctant to tell your closest confidant in life.

Remember, doctors too often misdiagnose dementia. Once the symptoms of these deadly dementias set in, you need to see your doctor, provide them with all the information about your problem, and help the specialists reach the correct diagnosis.

Because no tests exist for most dementias, doctors order tests and go through a process of elimination until reaching a diagnosis based on the symptoms you report. The more information you provide, the better the chance of a quick and accurate diagnosis.

Adopt healthy lifestyle choices to prevent dementia when possible, but the next best option is to diagnose it early, to confront it head-on, and take steps to slow the disease. Once dementia hits, it's often possible to postpone the advanced stages. If you've seen a loved one inflicted with dementia, you understand how precious a year, a month, a week, or day is once the storm aims at you or a loved one.

Prolonging life in late-stage dementia without a cure amounts to cruel and unusual punishment, but patients, families, and doctors must do everything possible to extend quality of life while possible.

Make certain you have a doctor who believes in prevention and natural cures, but also remember you need their expertise concerning the best that modern medicine offers.

Be Your Nurse!

If you have a loved one, be each other's nurse. If not, be your nurse.

It's more important than ever for you to monitor your blood pressure and make notes of health issues as they arise. We don't go to the doctor every time we develop a symptom or don't feel well, but it's important to keep a medical journal. Write an outline of the problems you experience between visits.

Too often, we march into the physician's office and don't provide a full or accurate representation of our problem. For instance, if you track your blood pressure, you can furnish a pattern rather than a onetime reading. You can also perhaps attribute pikes in your blood pressure to stress taking place in your life.

You should also track other symptoms. Providing thorough information helps doctors eliminate multiple diseases with similar symptoms. When you document all or most of the symptoms that have led to the visit, you provide a competent doctor a clearer picture to develop a hypothesis. These previous unrelated symptoms might help your physician make more sense of what prompted the appointment.

Otherwise, your physician might order the wrong tests or prescribe the wrong drugs. For issues of the brain, you can't be shy or embarrassed about providing your physician with a full portrayal of your problems and symptoms.

Although still stigmatized in some circles, mental illnesses are just as real, and the sufferers are no more the blame, than physical disorders. While we must do everything in our power to avoid or slow mental or physical maladies, the last thing we need to do is embarrass those who are already suffering.

Two Dementia Series

The laborious task to document the primary dementias began as a fifty-page Alzheimer's overview. Two editions later, the 50-page Alzheimer's book turned into 400 pages.

One of the first lessons taught Alzheimer's is only one of the hundreds of diseases responsible for dementia. With inadequate testing, similar symptoms, and other handicaps, the medical community often misdiagnoses the other dementias for Alzheimer's.

My focus broadened from Alzheimer's to a dozen dementias. The only way to make any sense of Alzheimer's or dementia was to study all the primary dementias.

I worked with several neurologists and researchers over the next couple of years and hit every medical library I could hit in person or available online.

After an extensive review, I wrote the first book covering the 15 most prevalent dementia types, which provided the groundwork for two updated dementia series.

The associated *Dementia Types, Symptoms, Stages, & Risk Factors, series* expands the collection by adding amyotrophic lateral sclerosis (ALS), early-onset Alzheimer's disease, amyotrophic lateral sclerosis, corticobasal syndrome, and progressive supranuclear palsy.

Two Dementia Series

Not counting mixed dementia, there are nineteen primary dementia types, which two groundbreaking series covers.

Dementia Types, Symptoms, Stages, & Risk Factors series

1. _Dementia with Lewy Bodies_
2. _Parkinson's Disease Dementia_
3. _Corticobasal Syndrome_
4. _Typical Alzheimer's Disease_
5. _Posterior Cortical Atrophy_
6. _Down Syndrome with Alzheimer's_
7. _Limbic-predominant Age-related TDP-43 Encephalopathy (LATE)_
8. _Early-onset Alzheimer's_
9. _Behavioral Variant Frontotemporal Dementia_
10. _Progressive Supranuclear Palsy_
11. _Nonfluent Primary Progressive Aphasia_
12. _Logopenic Progressive Aphasia_
13. _Cortical Vascular Dementia_
14. _Binswanger Disease_
15. _Normal Pressure Hydrocephalus_
16. _Huntington's Disease_
17. _Korsakoff Syndrome_
18. _Creutzfeldt-Jakob Disease_
19. _Amyotrophic Lateral Sclerosis_

*Not a dementia type, but a combination, mixed dementia is the 20th category important in dementia discussions.

Any disease leading to associated symptoms is a dementia type. The series breaks medical ground by covering the dementias responsible for over 99% of dementia cases.

Dementia Overview Series

The second series focuses on all the primary dementia types or breaks them down as groups.

2020 Dementia Overview Series

1. _Dementia Types, Symptoms, & Stages_
2. _Lewy Body/Parkinsonism Dementias_
3. _Vascular Dementia_
4. _Frontotemporal Dementia (FTD)_
5. _Alzheimer's Related Dementias_
6. _Prevent or Slow Dementia_

The Best Science in Everyday Language

The text in both series contains American, Australian, British, and other English. I write in American English, but the research comes from the best studies worldwide. Quotes from the UK, Australia, and other English-speaking countries depend on the local dialect. For integrity, I do not edit quotes.

The books include facts and science as they exist. As much as possible, we replace medical jargon with everyday language.

Having explained the series, let's discuss dementia.

I. DEMENTIA

In this section, we discuss dementia.

Dementia is not a disease but a medical condition. Hundreds of diseases and disorders lead to dementia, but percentage-wise, almost all dementia falls under 19 primary dementia categories.

This series is the first to cover all 19 primary dementia types.

In this chapter, we answer the following questions:

- What is dementia?
- What are the 19 primary dementias?
- How prevalent is dementia?
- Who is most likely to get dementia?
- What are the financial costs to individuals, the U.S., and worldwide?

Once we answer these questions and provide a dementia overview, we turn our attention to the subject matter for the rest of the book.

Let's begin by answering the question: What is dementia?

Chapter 1: WHAT IS DEMENTIA?

For centuries, when one got dementia, people described the person in terms like "gone mad," or "lost their mind," or "crazy," or another derogatory term that missed the mark.

While most dementia types attack cognitive skills and cause behavioral disorders, the person is no less a victim than a cancer patient.

Whereas cancer attacks cells and organs, dementia destroys brain neurons.

The brain is complex. One-hundred billion neurons use over 100 trillion synapses and about 100 neurotransmitters to send all the signals to other parts of the brain, organs, and parts throughout the body, allowing us to think, reason, walk, talk, breathe, and do all that makes us human.

When fed, protected, and healthy, neurons perform magic.

The different dementias attack the brain and destroy the communication network responsible for everything our body does. By attacking different parts of the brain, the dementia types cause different disorders.

Let's see how some of the most prestigious American and global medical organizations define Dementia.

Alzheimer's Association Definition

Let's begin with the Alzheimer's Association:

> *Dementia is an overall term for diseases and conditions characterized by a decline in memory, language, problem-solving, and other thinking skills that affect a person's ability to perform everyday activities. Memory loss is an example. Alzheimer's is the most common cause of dementia[1].*

Dementia is to Alzheimer's, dementia with Lewy bodies,

Parkinson's dementia, vascular and the other dementia types what Asia is to China, India, North Korea, South Korea, and the rest of Asia. Alzheimer's is the most prevalent dementia, but each type devastates, and most are death sentences.

Let's turn to the National Institute on Aging (NIH) and see how they define dementia.

National Institute on Aging (NIH)

The National Institute on Aging (NIH) funds many studies and provides researchers invaluable data. How do they define dementia?

> *Dementia is the loss of cognitive functioning – thinking, remembering, and reasoning – and behavioral abilities to such an extent that it interferes with a person's daily life and activities. These functions include memory, language skills, visual perception, problem-solving, self-management, and the ability to focus and pay attention. Some people with dementia cannot control their emotions, and their personalities may change. Dementia ranges in severity from the mildest stage, when it is just beginning to affect a person's functioning, to the most severe stage, when the person must depend completely on others for basic activities of living[2].*

One of the most important things a person and their loved ones can do when diagnosed with dementia; enjoy what quality time remains.

Early diagnosis, medication, and lifestyle changes can slow the disease and extend quality life. From the point of diagnosis, make the most of each good day or moment.

Let's see how the international community defines dementia.

Alzheimer's Society UK

The Alzheimer's Society is perhaps the UK's most

prestigious Alzheimer's organization. They define dementia:

The word 'dementia' describes a set of symptoms that may include memory loss and difficulties with thinking, problem-solving or language. These changes are often small to start with, but for someone with dementia they have become severe enough to affect daily life. A person with dementia may also experience changes in their mood or behaviour[3].

Let's see how the World Health Organization (WHO) defines dementia.

World Health Organization (WHO)

The World Health Organization (WHO) works with global medical organizations and provides researchers a wealth of information. How does WHO define dementia?

Dementia is a syndrome – usually of a chronic or progressive nature – in which there is deterioration in cognitive function (i.e. the ability to process thought) beyond what might be expected from normal ageing. It affects memory, thinking, orientation, comprehension, calculation, learning capacity, language, and judgement. Consciousness is not affected. The impairment in cognitive function is commonly accompanied, and occasionally preceded, by deterioration in emotional control, social behaviour, or motivation[4].

The four organizations provide similar definitions, each emphasizing different points, but none contradicting the others.

Each organization confirms dementia is a broad neurological disorder. Hundreds of pathologies such as Alzheimer's leads to dementia, but 19 primary types cause about 99% of dementia cases. Dementia attacks the brain and causes memory decline, behavior disorders, motor decline, language deterioration, and most types are incurable.

If doctors diagnose you with dementia, you must get past the shock. Time is moving against you, so make the most of it.

As the Alzheimer's Society points out, the symptoms are minor in the beginning. Get your affairs in order, enjoy loved ones, and take part in as many activities as you desire and are able. To some extent, this is your farewell tour. Take advantage!

The disease will stop you or a loved one later, so do not stop living your life in the early stages.

Let's next examine the 19 primary dementia types.

Chapter 2: WHAT ARE THE 19 PRIMARY DEMENTIAS?

Hundreds of medical conditions lead to dementia, but 19 causes up to 99% of cases.

Each dementia type is devastating, most are fatal, and the first symptoms to death is a challenging, heartbreaking, soul-crushing experience. Dementia robs the personalities and functionality of marvelous people a little at a time until they no longer resemble the person they've always been.

19 Dementia Types

This chapter divides the 19 primary dementias into six categories. The first group includes dementias related to Lewy body or Parkinsonism dementia. The second consists of Alzheimer's-related dementia. In the third, we focus on primary progressive aphasia dementias. The fourth contains vascular dementias. The fifth category encompasses the remaining dementias and is called *other dementias*.

Lewy Body/Parkinsonism Related Dementias

1. *Dementia with Lewy Bodies*
2. *Parkinson's Disease Dementia*
3. Corticobasal Syndrome

Alzheimer's Related Dementias

4. Typical Alzheimer's Disease
5. *Posterior Cortical Atrophy*
6. *Down Syndrome with Alzheimer's*
7. *Limbic-predominant Age-related TDP-43 Encephalopathy (LATE)*
8. Early-onset Alzheimer's

Frontotemporal Lobar Degeneration Related Dementias

9. *Behavioral Variant Frontotemporal Dementia*
10. Progressive Supranuclear Palsy

Primary Progressive Aphasia Related Dementias

11. *Nonfluent Primary Progressive Aphasia (nfvPPA)*
12. Logopenic Progressive Aphasia (LPA)

Vascular Dementia

13. *Cortical Vascular Dementia*
14. *Binswanger Disease*

Other Dementias

15. *Normal Pressure Hydrocephalus*
16. *Huntington's Disease*
17. *Korsakoff Syndrome*
18. *Creutzfeldt-Jakob Disease*
19. Amyotrophic Lateral Sclerosis

Chapter 3: WHO IS MOST LIKELY TO GET DEMENTIA?

In this chapter, we explore who is most likely to get dementia. Most know people with dementia are old, but some people are born with dementia, others get it as infants, and the disease attacks people in every age group.

There are risk factors that affect everybody. Examples include a poor diet, lack of exercise, diabetes, obesity, high blood pressure, and factors under and beyond our control.

In this chapter, we focus on risk factors affecting specific groups of people who suffer higher rates.

The research pointed to age, race, and sex, where dementia seems to discriminate. Let's review the science for each.

Age

Age is the obvious risk factor. We know because of science and our observations.

So associated with the elderly, many believe dementia only strikes older people. However, dementia strikes all ages and demographics, including newborns and infants.

According to Stanford University Medical School, "The risk of Alzheimer's disease, vascular dementia, and several other dementias goes up significantly with advancing age[5]."

None of us enjoy aging. We must work harder and harder to slow aging, and no matter how well we do, none of us will make it much past 100 years. The better we take care of ourselves, the higher chance we have of living a quality life into our eighties or nineties.

Remember, aging does not destroy our cognitive abilities. Bad habits do! I stress this point because each of us can slow the aging process through healthy habits.

As people age, however, our dementia risks increase.

A Journal of Neurology, Neurosurgery, & Psychiatry study concluded[6]:

> *In the age group 65–69 years, there are more than two new cases per 1000 persons every year. This number increases almost exponentially with increasing age, until over the age of 90 years, out of 1000 persons, 70 new cases of dementia can be expected every year.*

As we stress in our book on prevention, there is actual age and real age. We determine one's actual age by the day and year born, whereas weight, blood pressure, blood sugar, cholesterol, diet, how often you work out, and several other important factors govern our real age.

Unless genes or an accident prevents us, our real age should be lower than our actual age. Those who practice bad habits, however, raise their real age ten years or more than their actual age.

When our real age is lower than our actual age, we lower our risks for dementia and other diseases. When our real age is higher than our actual age, we increase risks for dementia, heart disease, cancer, and all major diseases.

Let's next review if race plays a role in dementia.

Race

African Americans and blacks in western countries suffer more than their share of racism.

The United States has abused too many citizens since its creation, but none more than Native Americans and African Americans.

But, does dementia also discriminate against them?

According to AARP, African Americans are 64% more likely to get dementia than non-Hispanic whites[7].

Kaiser Permanente Study

Researchers in another study examined data from 274,000 Kaiser Permanente patients over 14 years. They found the highest rate of dementia for African Americans and Native Americans[8].

Dementia Risk Per 1,000 People

27 African Americans

22 Native Americans

20 Latinos and Pacific Islanders

19 White Americans

15 Asian-Americans

Does dementia love Asian and European-Americans and hate African and Native-Americans?

Dementia is as evil as the worst bigot, but dementia is not a bigot.

African Americans experience higher rates of diabetes. African Americans and Native Americans suffer a higher level of stress, poverty, and disenfranchisement. Both cultures also struggle with their people's history in European-America and endure a greater level of bigotry and more obstacles to succeeding in modern America.

On the flip side, Asian Americans and whites have lower obesity and diabetes rates, eat a more balanced diet, faceless bigotry, are more affluent, educated, and successful in modern America.

We need more studies to confirm the exact causes of higher dementia incidence in the African and Native American populations. Higher stress and diabetes in their communities are prime suspects.

Jennifer Manly, Columbia University, Taub Institute for Research on Alzheimer's disease, and Aging Brain spoke to Reuters about the inequities.

> *There are huge disparities in dementia that are confronting this nation, and this will translate into an enormous burden on families if we don't address this. We need to prioritize research that uncovers the reasons for these disparities and more research should include racially and ethnically diverse people[9].*

Are African British at a greater risk for Dementia?

In the United Kingdom, black women are 25% more likely than white women, and black men 28% more likely than white men to get dementia[10].

Reluctance to Take Part in Dementia Studies

African Americans and Native Americans are also less trustful of studies. Too often in the past, a bigoted establishment treated African Americans and Native Americans like lab rats.

The awful past makes the average African American reluctant to take part in studies that might help us figure out how to lower the rates.

Native Americans are also distrustful of the United States government and the "white man's studies," as one group from the Cherokee Reservation in North Carolina told me.

I understand both ethnic groups' skepticism. As somebody with ancestors who died and survived the Trail of Tears, and who married a black woman (30+ years), nobody must convince me of the tainted American history. I have read about the past and viewed enough with my own eyes to know the sins of America's past, either haunt or still torment today.

But, the Studies are Necessary!

I call on African Americans and Native Americans to take part in dementia studies. The studies today have greater safeguards than the past and face much more scrutiny.

Dementia is a death sentence!

Worse than the average killer, never content to kill and move on, dementia is a sadist. Dementia destroys the mind and body, little by little, robbing one's personality, dignity, mind, body, and everything that makes a person unique.

If African Americans and Native Americans refuse to participate in dementia studies, fatal neurological disorders will continue to strike them worse than other ethnic groups.

Please consider two facts.

If you do not have dementia, researchers do not subject you to drug trials but accumulate data to determine which habits increase and decrease one's risks.

If doctors diagnose you with dementia, trials represent your last best chance to win what is otherwise a losing battle.

What Role does Poverty Play?

Although not listed as a dementia risk factor, poverty increases one's risk for almost every significant disease. Those at the bottom must worry where the next meal is coming, if somebody might mug (or kill) them when leaving the house, and a laundry list of stress the average citizen seems oblivious.

Beller Health calls for more research to determine if Native American, African American, and African British citizens have higher dementia rates as a general population, or if poverty drives these numbers. We need to know whether the number also applies to middle-and upper-class African Americans and Native Americans who eat healthily, exercise, do not abuse alcohol, avoid tobacco, and do not abuse prescription or illicit drugs.

Native American, African American, and African British citizens suffer a higher percentage of poverty than other demographics in the US and UK.

Rather than race, such factors as poverty, bigotry, and lack of opportunities might drive these numbers.

I reached out to several organizations, including the VA, to conduct a large-scale study to determine what role poverty plays in dementia. Most organizations greeted my request with enthusiasm, and I hope one or more soon back the study.

All we know for certain is poverty in the industrial world causes a much greater level of stress and other hardships than the rest of the population. WHO reported that about 60% of dementia cases occur in the poorest half of countries[11].

Age and ethnicity are dementia risk factors. What about sex?

Sex

Dementia strikes older people, African Americans, Native Americans, and African British in greater numbers than the rest of the population. Does one's gender increase or decrease one's odds?

How Many Women have Dementia?

According to the Alzheimer's Association, women represent two-thirds of people living with Alzheimer's, and 13 million women suffer dementia or are caring for somebody who does[12].

Of the 820,000 people living with dementia in the UK, females account for 61 percent[13].

Of the 50 million people living with dementia worldwide[14], women represent 65 percent[15].

Key points:

- Women represent two-thirds of Alzheimer's cases.
- Females account for 65% of dementia cases.

Is dementia just another woman-hating predator?

Does Alzheimer's & Most Dementia Strike Women in Greater Numbers?

While the two key numbers suggest dementia is a rampaging woman-abusing murderer, the answer is not so simple.

While women represent two-thirds of Alzheimer's cases and 65% of dementia cases, there are 19 primary dementia types.

Some dementias attack men in greater numbers and much harder than females. The dementias we know attack men in greater ratios include[16]:

- Parkinson's dementia (Lewy body dementia)
- Dementia with Lewy bodies (Lewy body dementia)
- Post-Stroke dementia (Vascular dementia)
- Multi-infarct dementia (Vascular dementia)
- Binswanger Disease(Vascular dementia)
- Normal pressure hydrocephalus
- Behavioral variant frontotemporal dementia
- Primary Progressive Aphasia (Frontotemporal dementia)
- Chronic traumatic encephalopathy
- HIV-related cognitive impairment
- Amyotrophic lateral sclerosis

From the data about the 19 primary dementias, at least eleven attack men in greater numbers. Data is not available for Creutzfeldt-Jakob disease, Wernicke-Korsakoff Syndrome, LATE, and Down syndrome with Alzheimer's disease. The remaining dementias strike both genders in similar numbers.

When the authorities release more information, we will update this section.

If a minimum of 11 of 19 dementia types strike men in greater numbers than women, how can 68% of people living with dementia be women?

Alzheimer's accounts for 60-80% of dementia, and two-thirds of people with Alzheimer's are women.

When we say dementia attacks, women, 65% to 35% men, we distort the picture. I call on the medical community to provide greater clarity. More precise, we should warn women to represent two-thirds of total Alzheimer's cases, but stress a minimum of 11 of 19 dementia types strike men in greater numbers.

Treating dementia and Alzheimer's as interchangeable terms is misleading. There are 19 primary dementias and 11 or more attack men in greater numbers. If we exclude Alzheimer's and focus on the other 18 primary dementia types, they attack men by far greater percentages.

With that stipulation, let's explore why Alzheimer's and some dementias attack women more than men.

Why Does Alzheimer's & Dementia Strike Women in Greater Numbers Than Men?

In part, unique burdens & responsibilities explain the disparity.

Women still fight today for equality. Like Native Americans, African Americans, and African British, the average woman carries burdens; the average man is clueless.

To be a woman, one fights for equality from birth in a "man's world," as the song and tradition attest. Among things unique to women:

- Menstrual cycles (ranging from mild to horrendous)
- Childbirth
- Menopause

Being a guy is also difficult, but there's no denying women are born with unique responsibilities and burdens.

As an aunt once retorted, if they live long enough, every woman suffers menstrual cycles until menopause "tortures it out."

Women Live Longer

Women outlive men in the United States and worldwide.

Worldwide, the average man lives to age 69.8, while the average woman lives 74.2 years[17]. These are the average numbers, so they fluctuate from region to region and country to country.

Let's see how these numbers compare to the United States.

American Comparisons

The CDC reports the average American male lives 76 years, compared to the average American woman who lives 81 years[18].

Why Do Women Live Longer Than Men?

Although women live longer, this might result because more men abuse alcohol, tobacco, and drugs, get less sleep, work in more hazardous jobs, suffer greater casualties in war, and take unnecessary risks.

The lead author of a study published in the *British Medical Journal*, Australian neuropsychiatrist Richard Cibulskis, confirmed some of my suspicions.

Men are much more likely to die from preventable and treatable non-communicable diseases, such as {ischemic} heart disease and lung cancer, and road traffic accidents[19].

Global population expert, Dr. Perminder Sachdev, confirmed my other suspicions in an interview with *Time*.

"Men are more likely to smoke, drink excessively and be overweight," Sachdev said. "They are also less likely to seek medical help early, and, if diagnosed with a disease, they are

31

more likely to be non-adherent to treatment." Sachdev also pointed out, "men are more likely to take life-threatening risks and to die in car accidents, brawls or gunfights[20]."

Although nature perhaps installed a natural order to preserve the female population, men's reckless nature might account for the five years difference in life expectancy between the genders.

It will interest to see if the numbers change as more women become more like men. Women are assuming greater roles in war, law enforcement, and other areas where even men with healthy habits have fallen. As the societal lines between men and women blur, the difference in life expectancy should fall.

In all honorable fields of life, women should go for it. Never has there been a better time to prove the equality of the sexes.

As far as men's bad habits, my hope is women continue to show better judgment and exercise greater restraint. Women will never prove their equality by emulating men's worse habits or trying to outdo us in the stupid department.

The best men and women rise on similar foundations. However, the worst men and women also share a foundation. My hope for humans getting our act together soon hinges on the average woman being better than the average man.

Love yourselves for your unique feminine qualities. Be equal, but please do not confuse out-drinking, out-smoking, out-drugging, acting more reckless, and stupid than men with being equal. We need fewer men like that, not more women!

Chapter 4: DEMENTIA COSTS & PREVALENCE

In this chapter, we review dementia prevalence and costs to governments, the world, caregivers, and patients.

How Many People Worldwide Suffer Dementia?

According to the World Health Organization (WHO), over 50 million people suffer dementia worldwide, with 10 million new cases each year[21].

How Many Americans Have Dementia?

In the United States, 5.8 million Americans live with dementia[22], with Alzheimer's representing 70% of cases.

Let's check the UK dementia numbers.

How Many People in The UK Have Dementia?

According to the Alzheimer's Society, 850,000 people in the UK live with dementia[23].

Alzheimer's Society reports that about 70% of those living in UK care homes suffer dementia.

The numbers show Americans, British, and global citizens suffering high rates of dementia. Let's see which countries' dementia strikes the hardest.

Which Countries Have the Highest Dementia Rate?

Per World Atlas, the following ten countries suffer the highest dementia rate of deaths per 100,000 people[24]:

1. Finland
2. USA
3. Canada
4. Iceland
5. Sweden
6. Switzerland
7. Norway
8. Denmark
9. The Netherlands
10. Belgium

As we review the list, per population, dementia strikes Americans in greater numbers than any country but Finland.

Why?

There are several explanations:

- Over two-thirds of Americans are obese or overweight.
- The other countries on the list also suffer higher obesity levels than most countries not on the list.
- Because of weight issues, the countries in question suffer high rates of diabetes and high blood pressure, both dementia risk factors.
- Americans consume more prescription drugs than people worldwide. While there is no data to confirm, I suspect the other countries on the list also have greater access and use more prescription drugs than poorer countries.

- They load the western diet with salt, sugar, and white processed flours.
- The average person in western countries lives longer than those in poorer nations.
- We will add other factors once data becomes available.
- People live longer in these countries than most not on the list (the older one lives, the greater the dementia risk)

Another explanation is more misdiagnosis and no-diagnosis in poorer countries around the world. Obesity and other risk factors are also less of a problem in developing countries.

I recommend global researchers compare the ten countries on this list. By viewing the similarities between the ten, we might better pinpoint the cause for Alzheimer's and the other dementias.

If we can figure out what the citizens from the ten nations are doing wrong, we can find the cause and means of preventing dementia. While I pointed to some of the most obvious risk factors, the most important common risk factor from the ten nations might be something unexpected.

Let's now examine dementia costs.

Dementia Costs

In this chapter, we analyze dementia costs. We examine the United States and global costs, then provide estimated costs per family.

What Does Dementia Cost the United States?

More than the entire economies of Finland and 166 other countries, dementia costs the United States $277 billion per year.

What Does Dementia Cost Worldwide?

Getting credible global numbers proves difficult, if not

impossible, in any medical research. Often, the best source is the World Health Organization (WHO). They collect data from around the world and are an essential source for medical researchers.

Getting accurate dementia numbers in richer countries is difficult. In the United States and the UK, black people hesitate to take part in dementia studies or to seek medical attention for symptoms.

In richer countries, there are still too many misdiagnoses.

Thus, if we cannot get ironclad numbers in the United States, the United Kingdom, and the industrial nations, the task proves even more difficult for developing countries.

If the United States and the United Kingdom have difficulty convincing black citizens to seek medical attention for dementia symptoms, the third world faces even greater obstacles.

In the third world, most areas do well to offer their citizens basic medical care. With no urine or blood test, many regions lack resources for CAT scans, MRIs, and other expensive imaging equipment to make a diagnosis.

Without urine or blood tests, diagnosing dementia costs more than low-income people with inadequate or no insurance can afford in the richest countries.

In the United States and industrial nations, doctors often misdiagnose the other 19 primary dementias for Alzheimer's or each other.

Expecting doctors in many third world nations to diagnose dementia with inferior or no equipment is to expect miracles. If it overwhelms medical professionals in the wealthier nations, we often expect third world doctors to perform miracles. What amazes is they often do!

However, no matter how well the average third world doctor treats typical medical conditions, even if trained, impoverished circumstances deny them the necessary equipment to diagnose dementia early, if at all. My comments are not criticism.

The average doctor's job is not to diagnose or treat

dementia, but they must recognize symptoms and refer the patient to neurologists. Primary care physicians are the first line of defense.

North, south, east, west, dementia overwhelms the medical community.

Having discussed the limitations, let's examine the data. While the numbers are ballpark figures, landing in the park is the keystone to estimation. In most cases, the real numbers are much higher.

According to the *World Alzheimer's Report,* global dementia costs a minimum of $1 trillion per year, and experts predict it will reach $2 trillion by 2030 if we find no cure[25].

Authorities should release new numbers over the next year, and we will update this section.

The *Alzheimer's Report* global cost estimations do not include informal care costs; another reason we consider the estimates conservative.

The Alzheimer's Report concluded:

> *Direct medical care costs account for roughly 20% of global dementia costs, while direct social sector costs and informal care costs each account for roughly 40%. The relative contribution of informal care is greatest in the African regions and lowest in North America, Western Europe and some South American regions, while the reverse is true for social sector costs.*

Whatever the real up-to-date costs, we must take action to reduce the burden on individuals and nations. If we do not invest in independent research to develop an effective urine or blood test, cure, and vaccine for each dementia type, the costs will smother economies throughout the world. The costs will cripple developing countries and destabilize the wealthiest.

We have no choice but to invest more in dementia research. No matter which country you live, your economy, security, and the health of your nation rides on us finding a cure or vaccine.

As a scientist, I find it disturbing climate change and independent dementia research are not major priorities. Most governments, businesses, and individuals who can afford to fund dementia remain MIA in the war against dementia.

Before we conclude this section, let's examine the dementia statistics side-by-side in the table below.

DEMENTIA STATISTICS

This table focuses on the number of people with dementia and the number of deaths per 100,000 among the nations chosen for comparison.

NATION	# OF PEOPLE WITH DEMENTIA	DEMENTIA DEATHS PER 100,000 PEOPLE	TOTAL COSTS (US DOLLARS)
Australia	447,115	29.61	$15 billion
Brazil	1 million +	10.71	$16.45 billion
Canadian	747,000	37.30	$10.4 billion
China	16.93 million	19.87	$69 billion
France	1.2 million	30.84	$37.91 billion
Germany	1.5 million	16.99	$57.57 billion
India	4 million	14.57	$28.38 billion
Italy	1.4 million	19.81	$29.96 billion
Japan	4.6 million	7.22	$14.8 billion
Mexico	800,000	3.62	Not available
Spain	800.000+	29.23	$19.98 million
Netherlands	280,000	39.37	$4.44 million
United States	5.8 million	44.41	$290 billion
United Kingdom	850,000	49.18	$26.3 billion

Sources: World Health Rankings[26], Alzheimer's Europe[27], NATSIM[28], Alzheimer's Society[29], Brain Test[30]

Other sources cited in the chapter.

The table comes from my book 2020 Dementia Overview, which covers cost and prevalence among comparative nations in greater detail.

Let's next discuss the dementia costs for caregivers.

What Does Dementia Cost Volunteer Caregivers?

Although 41% make less than $50,000, American voluntary caregivers devote a minimum of 18.4 billion hours per year to dementia patients.

Worth $232 billion per year, we underrate the voluntary caregiving heroes in our fight against dementia. This total does not include lost wages for the voluntary caregiver.

According to the Northwestern Mutual C.A.R.E. Study, 67% of voluntary caregivers must cut their living to help pay for the patient's medical care, and 57% end up experiencing financial problems[31].

Adding to the costs of voluntary caregivers, they often end up sick themselves. Caring for loved ones with dementia bankrupts many.

In the early stages, the loved one can still perform most of their daily tasks but will require 24/7 care once the symptoms advance.

Imagine putting your life on hold for years to care, bathe, feed, protect, and take such a heavy load on your shoulders.

Millions of dementia families face the dilemma where the husband and wife both must work in most families to get by. You work as a couple to build stability in your own family, and then, boom, doctors diagnose one of you with dementia.

What Does Dementia Cost Dementia Patients?

When we say patient, past a certain stage in the disease, we refer to family or loved ones. A person who cannot perform daily tasks cannot manage finances, even if they have any left.

Too often, the costs drive entire families into bankruptcy because of dementia costs for a member.

Authorities estimate the average cost per dementia patient is $341,840, with families expected to cover 70 percent.

The costs devastate the average family in the industrial nations.

How are they supposed to afford it in developing countries where the average citizen makes less than one-thousand American dollars per year?

Dementia Recap

Although your dementia research has just begun, you now have a decent overview of Dementia.

In Chapter One, we explored dementia. We turned to several top dementia or medical organizations and compared their definitions.

Chapter two explained Alzheimer's is to dementia what China is to Asia. We listed the 19 dementias. They include:

1. *Dementia with Lewy Bodies*
2. *Parkinson's Disease Dementia*
3. Corticobasal Syndrome
4. Typical Alzheimer's Disease
5. *Posterior Cortical Atrophy*
6. *Down Syndrome with Alzheimer's*
7. *Limbic-predominant Age-related TDP-43 Encephalopathy (LATE)*
8. Early-onset Alzheimer's
9. *Behavioral Variant Frontotemporal Dementia*
10. Progressive Supranuclear Palsy
11. *Nonfluent Primary Progressive Aphasia*
12. Logopenic Progressive Aphasia
13. *Cortical Vascular Dementia*
14. *Binswanger Disease*
15. *Normal Pressure Hydrocephalus*
16. *Huntington's Disease*
17. *Korsakoff Syndrome*
18. *Creutzfeldt-Jakob Disease*
19. Amyotrophic Lateral Sclerosis

Although most the dementia types share similar symptoms, enough to cause misdiagnosis, each has its unique pathology and symptoms.

In chapter three, we explored dementia prevalence in the United States, the UK, and worldwide.

Chapter four examined who is most likely to get dementia. We found Native Americans (those who greeted the first Europeans), and black citizens in the United States and the UK are more likely to get dementia than their white or Asian counterparts.

We also explored the women to men ratio. Women represent two-thirds of Alzheimer's and over sixty percent of dementia cases. We pointed out the Alzheimer's figure skews the dementia numbers because men are more likely to get a minimum of 11 of the 19 primary dementia types.

Chapter four explored the US, UK, global, patient, family, and voluntary caregivers' dementia costs. The staggering numbers are almost as frightening as the medical disorder itself.

We borrowed the following table from *2020 Dementia Overview.*

Dementia Costs & Prevalence

NATION	# OF PEOPLE WITH DEMENTIA	DEMENTIA DEATHS PER 100,000 PEOPLE	TOTAL COSTS (US DOLLARS)
Australia	447,115	29.61	$15 billion
Brazil	1 million +	10.71	$16.45 billion
Canadian	747,000	37.30	$10.4 billion
China	16.93 million	19.87	$69 billion
France	1.2 million	30.84	$37.91 billion
Germany	1.5 million	16.99	$57.57 billion
India	4 million	14.57	$28.38 billion
Italy	1.4 million	19.81	$29.96 billion
Japan	4.6 million	7.22	$14.8 billion
Mexico	800,000	3.62	Not available
Spain	800.000+	29.23	$19.98 million
Netherlands	280,000	39.37	$4.44 million
United States	5.8 million	44.41	$290 billion
United Kingdom	850,000	49.18	$26.3 billion

Sources: World Health Rankings[32], Alzheimer's Europe[33], NATSIM[34], Alzheimer's Society[35], Brain Test[36]

The table comes from 2020 Dementia Overview, which covers cost and prevalence among comparative nations in greater detail.

After reviewing the conservative numbers, and factoring in an aging population, we concluded we must find a cure before it bankrupts millions of families and overwhelms nations.

Having explained the series and introduced dementia, let's discuss the 19 primary dementia types.

Chapter 5: 19 PRIMARY DEMENTIA TYPES

Why is it important to learn about the most prevalent dementias?

There are several reasons. One, the dementias share similar symptoms and—with no accurate testing—doctors often misdiagnose for one of a hundred or more other possibilities. Two, if a person gets one dementia, more often than not, they develop an overlapping second dementia type, known as mixed dementia. In some cases, three dementia types might develop in later stages.

The pathology, related-proteins, atrophy location, and the resulting symptoms determine dementia classifications.

The more we learn about dementia, dementia types, and subtypes grow.

We once thought of Alzheimer's disease as one sweeping neurological disorder, but now know there is typical Alzheimer's, behavior variant Alzheimer's, posterior cortical atrophy, Early-onset Alzheimer's, and the newest dementia category, LATE, previously misdiagnosed for typical Alzheimer's. If that is not complicated enough, there are 20-40 typical Alzheimer's types.

Depending on the pathology, the three primary progressive aphasia subtypes are either Alzheimer's or frontotemporal-related.

We know there is not one vascular dementia, but three: post-stroke dementia, multi-infarct dementia, and Binswanger disease.

There are two Lewy body dementias; Parkinson's disease dementia and dementia with Lewy bodies. There are also other Parkinson-related neurological disorders.

The series covers the 19 most prevalent dementia types. As noted, several are subtypes, but this work extends each equal status and inquiry

Besides breaking down the twenty most prevalent dementia types, we also discuss subtypes for each.

To reduce repetition, we divide the 19 dementias into the following sections.

Lewy Body/Parkinsonism Related Dementias

1. *Dementia with Lewy Bodies*
2. *Parkinson's Disease Dementia*
3. Corticobasal Syndrome

Alzheimer's Related Dementias

4. Typical Alzheimer's Disease
5. *Posterior Cortical Atrophy*
6. *Down Syndrome with Alzheimer's*
7. *Limbic-predominant Age-related TDP-43 Encephalopathy (LATE)*
8. Early-onset Alzheimer's

Frontotemporal Lobar Degeneration Related Dementias

9. *Behavioral Variant Frontotemporal Dementia*
10. Progressive Supranuclear Palsy

Primary Progressive Aphasia Related Dementias

11. *Nonfluent Primary Progressive Aphasia (nfvPPA)*
12. Logopenic Progressive Aphasia (LPA)

Vascular Dementia

13. *Cortical Vascular Dementia*
14. *Binswanger Disease*

Other Dementias

15. *Normal Pressure Hydrocephalus*
16. *Huntington's Disease*
17. *Korsakoff Syndrome*
18. *Creutzfeldt-Jakob Disease*
19. Amyotrophic Lateral Sclerosis

Let's shift the discussion to our book topic, frontotemporal related dementia.

II. FTD-RELATED DEMENTIAS

The series devotes books to two FTD-related dementias:

1. Behavioral Variant Frontotemporal Dementia
2. Progressive Supranuclear Palsy

The PPA subtypes also have FTD links, but we list them separate as PPA dementias.

Chapter 6: WHAT IS FRONTOTEMPORAL DEMENTIA?

Perhaps the fourth largest dementia category, frontotemporal dementia does not receive the headlines, nor research money as its more popular cousins: Alzheimer's, Vascular dementia, and Lewy body dementia.

FRONTOTEMPORAL DEMENTIA

Sometimes called Pick's disease, frontotemporal dementia begins as frontotemporal degeneration (FTD) and progresses to dementia symptoms.

Frontotemporal dementia attacks the front and side sections of the brain. A steady, progressive disease, frontotemporal dementia causes behavior changes (problems) and destroys the ability to process language.

To further define frontotemporal dementia, let's turn to other authorities.

Frontotemporal dementia affects "the frontal and temporal lobes of the brain (the front and sides) in particular." according to the National Health Service in the UK. "These parts of the brain are largely responsible for language and the ability to plan and organise, and are important in controlling behaviour[37]."

The UCSF Weill Institute for Neurosciences describes FTD:

> *Frontotemporal dementia (FTD) is a group of related conditions resulting from the progressive degeneration of the temporal and frontal lobes of the brain. These areas of the brain play a significant role in decision-making, behavioral control, emotion and language[38].*

Depending on the neurological damage to the brain's frontal, temporal, and insular lobes, FTD produces contrasting symptoms. The divergence also explains why there are two primary subtypes.

According to the NIH, the brain's frontal lobes serves many purposes, including[39]:

- Censoring social behavior
- Managing emotional responses
- Processing language and communication

When the protein deposits form in the frontal lobes, depending on the exact location, the result is behavioral variant frontotemporal dementia or primary progressive aphasia.

If social behavior and emotion are predominant symptoms, this indicates behavioral variant frontotemporal dementia.

Neurological damage resulting in language and communication disorders suggest primary progressive aphasia.

As dementia develops and the deposits spread, the symptoms might overlap between the two primary frontotemporal dementia types.

What Is the Difference Between FTD And FLTD?

Many view FTD and FLTD as synonymous. Are FTD and FLTD synonymous?

No.

Frontotemporal dementia (FTD) is a frontotemporal lobar degeneration (FTLD) subtype. According to Dr. E. Mohandas, Elite Mission Hospital, "Frontotemporal disorders are forms of dementia caused by a family of brain diseases known as frontotemporal lobar degeneration (FTLD)."

Just as frontotemporal dementia (FTD) is one of many dementias, FTD is one of several FLTD neurological disorders caused by damage to the frontal lobes.

Who has the highest frontotemporal dementia risks?

Who does Frontotemporal Dementia (FTD) Strike?

Genetics causes a third of frontotemporal dementia[40].

While rarer than Alzheimer's, Lewy body dementia, and Vascular dementia, Frontotemporal dementia strikes more people in their 40s than most dementias.

Frontotemporal dementia accounts for over 20% of early-onset dementia.

Whereas women are more likely to have Alzheimer's, and men Lewy body dementia, frontotemporal is an equal opportunity killer and has no gender preference.

Frontotemporal dementia strikes people under 20 and over 80, but the average age diagnosis is 54. While far less prevalent than Alzheimer's for ages 65 and over, frontotemporal dementia strikes at a similar pace as early-onset Alzheimer's in 40-65 age groups.

A study released in the *Journal of Neurology, Neurosurgery & Psychiatry* concluded that 3% of seniors over 85 suffer Frontotemporal dementia[41].

How many people have Frontotemporal Dementia (FTD)?

Authorities can only estimate the number because doctors often misdiagnose frontotemporal dementia for other psychiatric disorders such as Alzheimer's or Parkinson's disease. About 60,000 Americans suffer frontotemporal dementia, although the number would climb much higher if we had an accurate urine or blood test.

I view American numbers as dubious, and the global numbers do not exist, as authorities cannot provide even a ballpark number.

One key to dementias such as frontotemporal is to discover accurate urine or blood tests for early diagnosis. As things stand, we do not know if the diagnosis is correct unless they perform an autopsy once the patient dies.

What Age Does Frontotemporal Dementia (FTD) Strike?

Most cases strike people between ages 40 and 65, although it inflicts people as young as 20 and in their eighties[42]. The average age for those diagnosed with frontotemporal dementia is age 57, which is 13 years younger than age 70 for other dementia patients[43].

"These disorders are among the most common dementias that strike at younger ages," according to John Hopkins Medicine. "Symptoms typically start between the ages of 40 and 65, but FTD can strike young adults and those who are older[44]."

What Causes Frontotemporal Dementia (FTD)?

Too often for dementias, the official answer within the medical community is the cause remains unknown, and this applies to frontotemporal dementia (FTD).

If science cannot name the exact cause, what do we know?

Genetics causes a third of FTD incidents. The number is higher than most dementias, except for down syndrome with Alzheimer's and Huntington's disease, which genetics is 100% responsible.

However, this means two/thirds of FTD cases are not family related. Nor does having a parent with FTD a dementia sentence.

Frontotemporal dementia is a sporadic neurological disorder. According to the Association for Frontotemporal Degeneration, one is no more at risk for FTD if a parent has the disorder than if they do not[45].

"Researchers have linked certain subtypes of FTD to mutations on several genes," per the University of Rochester Medical Center. "Some people with FTD have tiny structures, called Pick bodies, in their brain cells. Pick bodies have an abnormal amount or type of protein[46]."

Frontotemporal dementia manifests by damaging brain cells in the brain's frontal and temporal lobes.

Three FTD-related Dementia Types

There are three FTD associated dementias.

1. Behavior-variant frontotemporal dementia (bvFTD)
2. Primary progressive aphasia (PPA)
3. Progressive supranuclear palsy (PSP)

The former causes behavioral changes while the latter attacks language skills. Behavior-variant first destroys emotion while primary progressive aphasia robs the ability to speak and interpret language.

According to *Neuroscience Research Australia*, "When the initial damage is in the frontal lobe (called behavioral-variant FTD), the main changes are in personality and behaviour. Individuals with damage predominantly in the temporal lobe (either progressive non-fluent aphasia or semantic dementia) lose the ability to speak or understand language[47]."

Frontotemporal dementia (FTD) patients often suffer bvFTD and one or more of the primary progressive aphasias (PPA).

In slow grueling steps, the duel threats strip the person's ability to function as a normal adult in society.

We list the PPA subtypes in a separate section, so let's focus on behavioral variant frontotemporal dementia (bvFTD) and progressive supranuclear palsy (PSP).

Chapter 7: WHAT IS bvFTD BEHAVIORAL VARIANT FRONTOTEMPORAL DEMENTIA?

Sometimes called Pick's disease, frontotemporal dementia begins as frontotemporal degeneration (FTD) and progresses to dementia symptoms.

Frontotemporal dementia attacks the front and side sections of the brain. A steady, progressive disease, frontotemporal dementia causes behavior changes (problems) and destroys the ability to process language.

To further define frontotemporal dementia, let's turn to other authorities.

Frontotemporal dementia affects "the frontal and temporal lobes of the brain (the front and sides) in particular," according to the National Health Service in the UK. "These parts of the brain are largely responsible for language and the ability to plan and organise, and are important in controlling behaviour[48]."

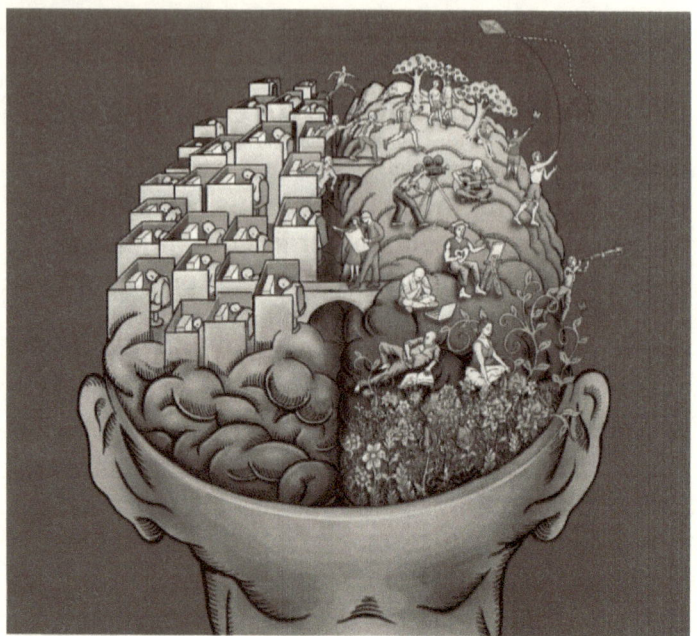

Right Brain[49]

Frontotemporal dementia stands out in a few ways. Genetics causes a third of incidents.

bvFTD strikes most people between ages 45 and 65, although it inflicts people as young as 20 and in their eighties[50]. The average age for those diagnosed with frontotemporal dementia is age 57, which is 13 years younger than age 70 for other dementia patients[51].

Frontotemporal dementia manifests by damaging brain cells in the brain's frontal and temporal lobes.

According to *Neuroscience Research Australia*, "When the initial damage is in the frontal lobe (called behavioral-variant FTD), the main changes are in personality and behavior. Individuals with damage predominantly in the temporal lobe (either progressive non-fluent aphasia or semantic dementia) lose the ability to speak or understand language[52]."

Behavioral Problems

According to Penn Frontotemporal degeneration Center, bvFTD: "is characterized by progressive atrophy (cell loss) in frontal and anterior temporal regions of the brain leading to alterations in complex thinking, personality, and behavior[53]."

The behavioral changes hurt family, friends, and associates. However, bvFTD patients suffer a wide range of emotional and behavioral disorders. While some behavior is unacceptable and loved ones and caregivers must help manage, the bvFTD patient has little or no control.

The UCSF Memory and Aging Center describes behavioral variant frontotemporal dementia.

People with behavioral variant frontotemporal dementia (bvFTD) often have trouble controlling their behavior. They may say inappropriate things or ignore other peoples' feelings. bvFTD may affect how a person deals with everyday situations. bvFTD can also affect language or thinking skills. Unfortunately, people with bvFTD rarely notice these changes[54].

Perhaps the most troubling aspect of the quote is the last sentence. The disease already chips away at the person's personality, but the victim remains oblivious.

The point illustrates the importance of loved ones monitoring each other's behavior.

Behavioral-variant frontotemporal dementia Prevalence

The most prevalent frontotemporal dementia, bvFTD, accounts for 50-70% of cases within the FTD family. If the 20% gap in possibilities gives pause, join the club.

Getting an exact number of FTD cases is impossible.

FTD Percentage of Dementia

The Association of Frontotemporal Degeneration estimates FTD totals 10-20% of dementia[55]. However, Stanford Medical School claims FTD represents 2-10% of dementia cases[56]. Other reputed authorities estimate the numbers 2-20%, some towards the high and others the low end.

NIH and those who control medical research funding sometimes neglect bvFTD because of other dementias such as Alzheimer's, Lewy body dementia, and vascular dementia strike more seniors 65 and older.

While I understand the logic of devoting most research money where it might help the most people, such thinking only works in theory, and sometimes not at all in practice.

As a man in my sixties, I want cures for disorders striking seniors, but I challenge suggestions we should not devote research money towards rarer disorders that strike young people in disproportionate numbers.

FTD Early Dementia Percentage

If we consider early-onset dementia even more devastating than late-onset dementia, we must view bvFTD and the FTD related dementias as significant.

Frontotemporal dementia strikes more people in their 40s than most dementias. Indeed, FTD is a leading cause of early-onset dementia. Frontotemporal dementia accounts for over 20% of early-onset dementia.

A *PubMed* study shows FTD accounts for 30.6% of early-onset dementia[57]. Exact percentages vary, but experts agree FTD is the second-leading cause of early-onset dementia, behind only Alzheimer's.

How many people have Frontotemporal Dementia?

Before I give a number, please note doctors often misdiagnose frontotemporal dementia for other psychiatric disorders such as Alzheimer's or Parkinson's disease. With that limitation, authorities estimate 60,000 Americans suffer frontotemporal dementia. However, the number would climb much higher if we had an accurate urine or blood test.

While a certain amount of malpractice occurs, like in any profession, I blame the majority of misdiagnoses on not having a blood or urine test.

Like the fictional Star Trek character, *Bones* used to retort: "I'm a doctor, not a miracle-worker, dammit!"

In real life, I would not blame the average general practitioner for throwing their arms up in the air and uttering the same line. Expecting a doctor to diagnose the various dementias and neurological disorders without urine or blood tests for most is as unrealistic as expecting a team of kayakers to win the Olympics without paddles.

Who does Frontotemporal Dementia Strike?

Genetics causes one-third of frontotemporal dementia[58].

Whereas women are more likely to have Alzheimer's, and men Lewy body dementia, frontotemporal is an equal opportunity killer and has no gender preference.

Frontotemporal dementia strikes people under 20 and over 80, but the average age diagnosis is 54. While far less prevalent than Alzheimer's for ages 65 and over, frontotemporal dementia strikes at a similar pace as early-onset Alzheimer's in 40-65 age groups.

A study released in the *Journal of Neurology, Neurosurgery & Psychiatry* concluded that 3% of seniors over 85 suffer Frontotemporal dementia[59].

One key to dementias such as frontotemporal is to discover accurate urine or blood test for early diagnosis. As things stand, we do not know if the diagnosis is correct unless they perform an autopsy once the patient dies.

bvFTD Recap

From the introduction, we know frontotemporal dementia (FTD) attacks the front and sides of the brain, the frontal, and temporal lobes.

We also know the frontal and temporal lobes are responsible for language, organizing, and behavior.

There are two types of FTD and primary progressive aphasia.

Other points to take from this section:

- 60,000 Americans suffer FTD
- There is no accurate test
- Doctors often misdiagnose FTD for Alzheimer's or other diseases
- FTD is one of the most prevalent dementias to strike people in their 40's or 50's in their prime

Closing thought

While behavioral variant frontotemporal dementia (bvFTD) represents most FTD cases, some develop both types. A person can also develop Alzheimer's or another dementia along with FTD, classified as mixed dementia.

Chapter 8: WHAT IS PROGRESSIVE SUPRANUCLEAR PALSY (PSP)?

Progressive means continuous severity. *Supranuclear* refers to the lesion cortical or superior to the brain's nucleus. *Palsy* suggests a weakness or paralysis, often associated with involuntary tremors.

The term *supranuclear palsy* indicates weakness or paralysis on one side of the body.

Also called Steele-Richardson-Olszewski syndrome, progressive supranuclear palsy is a neurological disorder that exhibits Parkinsonism symptoms such as balance, walking, speech, and other symptoms we soon discuss in greater detail.

In 1964, three scientists—John Steel, J. Clifford Richardson, and Jerzy Olszewski—published a study showing a divergence from typical Parkinson's disease.

Some still refer to their discovery as the Steel-Richardson-Olszewski syndrome, but most refer to the disorder as progressive supranuclear palsy.

Until 1964, neurologists recognized a case now and then but lumped them with Parkinson's disease. Cut the doctors some slack, however, as PSP and PD share some symptoms, and there was not a PSP category.

While it is tempting to bash doctors every time they misdiagnose dementia and sometimes justifiable, we must remember they cannot diagnose a disease not officially discovered.

As Dr. McKoy of Starship Enterprise used to grumble: "I'm a doctor, not a miracle worker, dammit!"

As with the fictional character, we often expect real-life doctors to do the impossible. Against great odds, the medical community produces seemingly miracles every day by overcoming near-impossible odds.

Not to excuse incompetence, but the best doctors also make mistakes with such limited tools. We cannot prevent dementia misdiagnosis by weeding out incompetent doctors. While the medical professional should weed out the unethical and incompetent, that alone will not prevent dementia misdiagnosis. Until we arm doctors with accurate blood or urine tests for each dementia, we expect the impossible.

Is there a PSP Cure?

As with most dementia-related diseases, there is no cure.

Diagnosing PSP poses challenges, leading to misdiagnoses or late diagnoses. A delayed diagnosis means delayed treatment, and misdiagnosis risks the wrong treatment. There are limited treatment options, which are too often not started early enough to slow the progression.

PSP Life Expectancy

Although PSP is not considered fatal, several later-stage symptoms often cause death, including choking, injuries, and pneumonia.

According to the NHS, from the time the symptoms manifest, the normal average PSP life range is 6-10 years[60].

How Many People Get Progressive Supranuclear Palsy (PSP)?

NIH estimates progressive supranuclear palsy inflicts six of every 100,000 people worldwide, and that 20,000 Americans live with PSP[61].

According to ASCE Neuron, PSP represents 1% of dementia[62].

Who Is Most Likely to Get Progressive Supranuclear Palsy (PSP)?

Progressive supranuclear palsy (PSP) attacks those over 60 in greater numbers than those younger. PSP also attacks men more often than women.

Medscape claims most people get PSP in their 50's and 60's, and the symptoms manifest a third of the time for people under sixty[63].

There is no genetic or family link in most PSP cases, although science links it to an abnormal tau protein buildup.

How Does Progressive Supranuclear Palsy (PSP) Differ from Parkinsons' Disease?

While PSP and PD share several symptoms, progressive supranuclear palsy differs from Parkinson's in several ways.

Progressive supranuclear palsy progresses faster than Parkinson's disease (PD).

Whereas Parkinson's patients often tilt their heads forward, somebody with PSP is more likely to tilt theirs backward. Eye movements remain normal in most PD patients but are abnormal in progressive supranuclear palsy patients. Swallowing and speech are more severe in PSP than PD. PSP often spares patients the Parkinson's associated tremors[64].

Another significant difference separating the dementias are different proteins. Alpha-synuclein is linked to Parkinson's, while the tau protein is associated with progressive supranuclear palsy.

Progressive Supranuclear Palsy Causes

Common for dementia and other neurological disorders, we do not yet know the exact cause of progressive supranuclear palsy (PSP). Science, however, links the rogue PSP related protein, tau[65].

If you've read much about Alzheimer's, you know about protein tau and the associated tangles. The MAPT gene in chromosome 17q21 produces tau[66].

TAU the Superhero

A high-soluble microtubule-related protein, the tau family, includes six isoforms, including 352-441 amino acids.

Regarding neurological disorders, protein is a superhero

turned villain. As superheroes, tau plays a vital role in the central nervous system by regulating the axonal transport of vesicles and stabilizing microtubules.

TAU Turned Villain

What causes the tau to turn rogue remains a mystery, but there is a pattern. Important protein turns abnormal and attacks the very structure it once built, maintained, or protected.

ASCE NEURON explains progressive supranuclear palsy:

> *The hallmark of PSP is the accumulation of abnormal deposits of the protein tau in nerve cells in the brain so that the cells do not function properly and eventually die. The appearance of deposits of the microtubule-associated tau protein termed 'neurofibrillary tangles' is a common feature of tauopathies that is shared with Alzheimer's disease. These neuronal tau deposits are known to be a major driver of neurodegeneration[67].*

Rogue tau protein causes 30-40% of Alzheimer's disease and links to a few other dementias, including progressive supranuclear palsy (PSP).

PSP Cortical Fibrillary Tangles

Although found in the spinal cord and central cortex, globose neurofibrillary tangles are more prevalent in the subcortical areas. PSP neurodegeneration occurs in the basal ganglia.

III. FTD-RELATED DEMENTIAS SYMPTOMS

FTD related dementias occur in the frontal and temporal lobes causing a variety of cognitive, behavior, language, visual, and motor disorders.

Chapter 9:
FRONTOTEMPORAL-RELATED DEMENTIA SYMPTOMS

Science must uncover FTD risk factors and causes, but we know much about the symptoms. To make it easier to grasp, we divide the symptoms into behavioral, cognitive, language and communication, and others.

Behavioral Symptoms

- Personality changes[68]
- Mood swings[69]
- More withdrawn and secluded than usual[70]
- Nervous and obsessive behavior, which includes rubbing hands, tapping feet, pacing the same stretch, mumbling or humming[71] that didn't exist before[72]
- Rude behavior considered out of character[73]
- Uninhibited[74]
- Irritated over trivial matters[75]
- Inflexible thinking[76]
- Lacks compassion and empathy[77]
- Less enthusiastic[78]

The above symptoms are associated with behavioral variant frontotemporal dementia (bvFTD) and are not the victim's fault. The neurological disorder causes a person to act out of character because of neuron damage in the brain's area responsible for censoring and processing thoughts required to behave according to societal norms.

Next, let's examine cognitive symptoms.

Cognitive Symptoms

- Needs reminders to do basic daily tasks[79]
- Distracted easier and more often than usual[80]
- Impaired judgment[81]
- Incapable of abstract thought[82]
- Evolving dependence[83]
- Deteriorating organizational skills[84]
- Memory issues (advanced stages)[85]

Cognitive symptoms somewhat resemble Alzheimer's, often causing misdiagnosis. Documenting full symptoms helps doctors order the correct tests and reduce the odds of misdiagnosing FTD for one of the other prominent dementias.

As frontotemporal dementia advances, it becomes less distinguishable from Alzheimer's. In the late stage, most dementia types resemble each other because damage to the brain spreads.

With no FTD test, doctors must diagnose the disorder through a process of elimination.

Let's move to language and communication symptoms.

Language And Communication Symptoms

- Diminished vocabulary[86]
- Repeats the same phrases over and over like stuck in a loop[87]
- Repeats what other people say[88]
- Misuses words, such as referring to plates as spoons, or dogs as cats[89]
- Inarticulate[90]
- Less conversational[91]

These symptoms are related to PPA and its three subtypes, which we soon cover in greater detail. I labeled the last category of FTD symptoms as others.

Other Symptoms

- Change in eating habits, including eating much more,

liking foods you always hated before[92]
- Deterioration of personal hygiene[93]

These symptoms are problematic for both frontotemporal dementia subtypes.

If you notice several uncharacteristic behaviors from the list in you or a loved one, see a neurologist at once. Document the symptoms you're experiencing, to enhance your physician's diagnosis.

No two patients develop exact frontotemporal dementia symptoms, as FTD uniquely strikes each. The smallest difference where FTD first attacks the brain produces a wide variety of symptoms. How the symptoms develop once somebody gets frontotemporal dementia also depends on the brain area affected and how fast FTD attacks.

When the listed symptoms appear, you or your loved one cannot see a competent doctor fast enough. While the medical community possesses no cures in their bag of tools, they can treat and slow symptoms, which extends the quality of life.

Until we find a cure, individuals must focus on how to prevent or slow dementia, and the medical community must treat symptoms with drugs and help the patient through a variety of physical, speech, and occupational therapy.

Instead of panicking, which is natural, the diagnosed and family must pull yourselves together and do what you can to make the most of what is left.

The person diagnosed and their loved ones must ask: **What is one more day, week, month, or year of quality time worth?**

I am not suggesting anybody neglect the many burdens the diagnosis brings on an individual and their closest loved ones.

Address future concerns, financial and otherwise. Create a Living Will, provide a trustworthy person the Power of Attorney, and get out in front of the coming storm while you can.

Figure out who will take care of you or a loved one when daily help becomes necessary. Understand such caregiving becomes a 24/7 job down the stretch.

The mentioned tasks and other steps are priorities, but prioritize extending the quality of life as long as possible. When we remove the medical, legal, and economic decisions, the most important thing is for everybody concerned to overcome the shock, hurt, and pain.

In the early stages, the symptoms are not usually severe enough to prevent somebody from carrying on much as usual. The challenge for you and your loved ones is to go on enjoying life while possible. Instead of dreading the coming storm, embrace the remaining possibilities.

Let's view the primary frontotemporal dementia (FTD) subtype, progressive supranuclear palsy (PSP).

Chapter 10: BEHAVIORAL VARIANT FRONTOTEMPORAL DEMENTIA (bvFTD) SYMPTOMS

In the image below, we are interested in the Frontal lobe and the Temporal lobe regions, the front and sides of the brain.

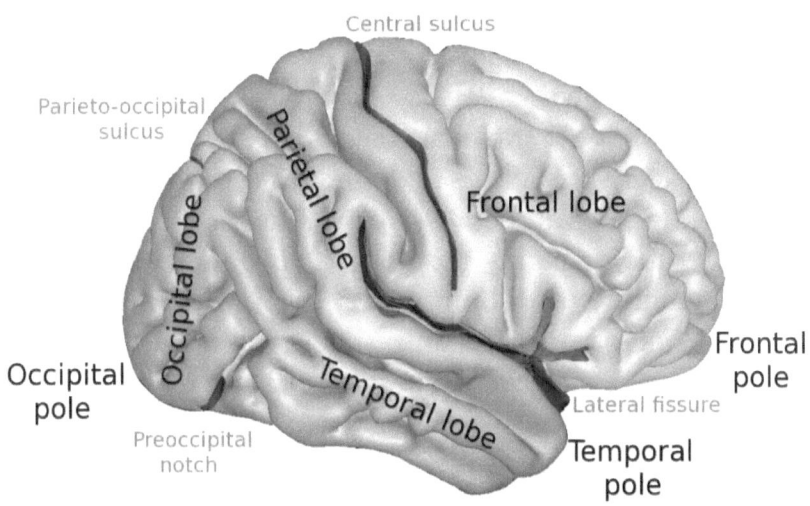

Posterior cortical atrophy[94]

While science must determine the risk factors and causes, we know much more about the symptoms of frontotemporal dementia:

- Behavioral changes[95]
- Change in eating habits, including eating much more, liking foods you always hated before[96]
- Deterioration of personal hygiene[97]

- Diminished vocabulary[98]
- Distracted easier and more often than usual[99]
- Irritated over trivial matters[100]
- Evolving dependence[101]
- Impaired judgment[102]
- Inarticulate[103]
- Incapable of abstract thought[104]
- Inflexible thinking[105]
- Lacks compassion and empathy[106]
- Less conversational[107]
- Less enthusiastic[108]
- Memory issues (advanced stages)[109]
- Muscle spasms[110]
- Misuses words, such as referring to plates as spoons, or dogs as cats[111]
- Mood changes[112]
- More withdrawn and secluded than usual[113]
- Needs reminders to do basic daily tasks[114]
- Nervous and obsessive behavior, which includes rubbing hands, tapping feet, pacing the same stretch, mumbling or humming[115] that didn't exist before[116]
- Deteriorating organizational skills[117]
- Repeats the same phrases over and over like stuck in a loop[118]
- Repeats what other people say[119]
- Rude behavior considered out of character[120]
- Uninhibited[121]

If you notice several uncharacteristic behaviors from the list in you or a loved one, see a neurologist at once. Write all the symptoms you're experiencing, to enhance your physician's diagnosis.

Let's break the symptoms down by category.

bvFTD Symptoms

To make it easier to grasp, we divide the symptoms into behavioral, cognitive, and others.

Behavioral Symptoms

- Personality changes[122]
- Mood swings[123]
- More withdrawn and secluded than usual[124]
- Nervous and obsessive behavior, which includes rubbing hands, tapping feet, pacing the same stretch, mumbling or humming[125] that didn't exist before[126]
- Rude behavior considered out of character[127]
- Uninhibited[128]
- Irritated over trivial matters[129]
- Inflexible thinking[130]
- Lacks compassion and empathy[131]
- Less enthusiastic[132]

The above symptoms are associated with behavioral variant frontotemporal dementia (bvFTD) and are not the victim's fault. The neurological disorder causes a person to act out of character because of neuron damage in the brain's area responsible for censoring and processing thoughts required to behave according to societal norms.

Next, let's examine cognitive symptoms.

Cognitive Symptoms

- Needs reminders to do basic daily tasks[133]
- Distracted easier and more often than usual[134]
- Impaired judgment[135]
- Incapable of abstract thought[136]
- Evolving dependence[137]

- Deteriorating organizational skills[138]
- Memory issues (advanced stages)[139]

Cognitive symptoms somewhat resemble Alzheimer's, often causing misdiagnosis. Documenting full symptoms helps doctors order the correct tests and reduce the odds of misdiagnosing bvFTD for one of the other prominent dementias.

As frontotemporal dementia advances, it becomes less distinguishable from Alzheimer's. In the late stage, most dementia types resemble each other because damage to the brain spreads.

With no FTD test, doctors must diagnose the disorder through a process of elimination.

Let's move to other symptoms.

Other Symptoms

- Change in eating habits, including eating much more, liking foods you always hated before[140]
- Deterioration of personal hygiene[141]

These symptoms are problematic for both frontotemporal dementia subtypes.

If you notice several uncharacteristic behaviors from the list in you or a loved one, see a neurologist at once. Document the symptoms you're experiencing, to enhance your physician's diagnosis.

No two patients develop exact frontotemporal dementia symptoms, as bvFTD uniquely strikes each. The smallest difference where FTD first attacks the brain produces a wide variety of symptoms. How the symptoms develop once somebody gets frontotemporal dementia also depends on the brain area affected and how fast bvFTD attacks.

When the listed symptoms appear, you or your loved one cannot see a competent doctor fast enough. While the medical community possesses no cures in their bag of tools, they can treat and slow symptoms, which extends the quality of life.

Until we find a cure, individuals must focus on how to

prevent or slow dementia, and the medical community must treat symptoms with drugs and help the patient through a variety of physical, speech, and occupational therapy.

Instead of panicking, which is natural, the diagnosed and family must pull yourselves together and do what you can to make the most of what is left.

The person diagnosed and their loved ones must ask: **What is one more day, week, month, or year of quality time worth?**

I am not suggesting anybody neglect the many burdens the diagnosis brings on an individual and their closest loved ones.

Address future concerns, financial and otherwise. Create a Living Will, provide a trustworthy person the Power of Attorney, and get out in front of the coming storm while you can.

Figure out who will take care of you or a loved one when daily help becomes necessary. Understand such caregiving becomes a 24/7 job down the stretch.

The mentioned tasks and other steps are priorities, but prioritize extending the quality of life as long as possible. When we remove the medical, legal, and economic decisions, the most important thing is for everybody concerned to overcome the shock, hurt, and pain.

In the early stages, the symptoms are not usually severe enough to prevent somebody from carrying on much as usual. The challenge for you and your loved ones is to go on enjoying life while possible. Instead of dreading the coming storm, embrace the remaining possibilities.

Chapter 11: PROGRESSIVE SUPRANUCLEAR PALSY SYMPTOMS

Progressive supranuclear palsy causes a wide range of behavior and mood problems. As with any neurological disorder causing behavior issues, this can be difficult for loved ones and caregivers.

However, you must remember the behavior is not the person's fault, but a neurological disorder destroys part of their mind. The frontal and temporal lobes are often involved with behavior and mood problems, which is why progressive supranuclear palsy lists in the frontotemporal degeneration family.

However, PSP related symptoms go well beyond the associated mood and behavior disorders to include a devastating attack on motor skills and muscle control.

NIH describes progressive supranuclear palsy symptoms.

The pattern of signs and symptoms can be quite different from person to person. The most frequent first symptom of PSP is a loss of balance while walking. Individuals may have unexplained falls or a stiffness and awkwardness in gait.

As the disease progresses, most people will begin to develop a blurring of vision and problems controlling eye movement. In fact, eye problems, in particular slowness of eye movements, usually offer the first definitive clue that PSP is the proper diagnosis. Individuals affected by PSP especially have trouble voluntarily shifting their gaze vertically (i.e., downward and/or upward) and also can have

76

trouble controlling their eyelids. This can lead to a need to move the head to look in different directions, involuntary closing of the eyes, prolonged or infrequent blinking, or difficulty in opening the eyes.

As NIH illustrates, progressive supranuclear palsy produces a wide range of symptoms. The symptoms start as young as forty, but not until the early sixties for most PSP patients.

To some extent, progressive supranuclear palsy is a combination of Parkinson's and behavioral frontotemporal dementia, attacking both the mind and the body.

Let's list the most common earlier stage symptoms.

PSP Symptoms

Progressive supranuclear palsy symptoms include:

- Apathetic
- Balance issues
- Behavior changes (reckless and flawed decision-making
- Blurred or double vision
- Falling (often backward)
- Irritable
- Major fatigue
- Moody
- Muscles discomfort
- Neck stiffness
- Personality changes
- Photophobia (bright lights sensitivity)
- Trouble looking up or down

PSP Symptoms Sources: National Health Services[142], National Institute of Neurological Disorders and Stroke[143]

We discuss progressive supranuclear palsy symptoms more in the symptoms section.

IV. FTD-RELATED DEMENTIAS STAGES

Let's now see how the FTD symptoms progress through stages.

Chapter 12: BEHAVIORAL VARIANT FRONTOTEMPORAL DEMENTIA (bvFTD) STAGES

There are seven stages to the general dementia category. Authorities offer different numbers for frontotemporal dementia. Some list three: mild, moderate, and severe. Others list five to seven. When using a seven stages model, the first stage is normalcy or no symptoms, while the seventh stage is the crippling period in the end. They are all variations of mild, moderate, and severe.

We use a four-stage model.

There are four stages to bvFTD (behavioral variant frontotemporal dementia).

1. Mild bvFTD
2. Moderate bvFTD
3. Severe bvFTD
4. Critical bvFTD

Stage 1: Mild bvFTD (behavioral variant frontotemporal dementia)

Cognitive impairment begins.

Mild bvFTD causes gray matter loss in the fronto paralimbic cortex and atrophy around the anterior cortical and subcortical[144].

In most people, the bvFTD symptoms begin mild and proceed slow but steady until a person demands 24/7 help in later stages.

In the mild bvFTD stage, a person is still fluent, remembers names, has normal comprehension, reading skills remain intact, and they suffer no reception issues.

Mild bvFTD causes aberrant behavior and personality changes.

- Apathetic
- Becomes anti-social
- Financial mismanagement
- Less interested in friends, family, and hobbies
- Impaired judgment
- Impulsive (inappropriate behavior, perhaps sexual, towards strangers, perhaps even break the law)
- Loss of empathy & sympathy for others
- Overeating (sugary foods)
- Planning problems

Let's view the clinical criteria for moderate bvFTD.

Stage 2: Moderate bvFTD

Any symptoms present in stage one now worsens.

- Apathetic
- Becomes anti-social
- Cannot manage household tasks
- Financial mismanagement
- Less interested in friends, family, and hobbies
- Impaired judgment
- Impulsive (inappropriate behavior, perhaps sexual, towards strangers, perhaps even break the law)
- Loss of empathy & sympathy for others
- Overeating (sugary foods)
- Planning problems

Slow and methodical, bvFTD marches through the brain, destroying or altering behavior, personality, memory, and overall health, the institutions of human life.

The person's cognitive skills decline in tiny steps and destroy, not in minutes, hours, days, or weeks, but over months and years.

In stage two, they will require supervision to engage in activities and perform household chores once done as second-nature.

Bathing, dressing, putting on shoes, and other personal duties grow difficult, if not impossible, in stage two.

Stage 3: Severe to Critical bvFTD

Stage one and two symptoms manifest slow and steady until causing severe behavioral, language, and memory decline. The severity level grows critical around the midpoint of stage three.

Stage 3: Severe to Critical bvFTD Symptoms

Symptoms from stages 1 and 2 show a steady decline until they reach stage three and become severe. And they will now suffer language difficulties and memory problems.

If the first two stages turned the world upside-down, stage three kicks and batters the world until it is no longer recognizable. Loved ones now view all the beautiful little things they once took for granted as godsends.

Stage 3 symptoms include:

- Aggressive
- Binge eating
- Compulsive cleaning
- Hoarding
- Overeating/overweight
- Unwanted, repetitious movements
- Unfocused
- Wandering
- Apathetic
- Becomes anti-social
- Cannot manage household tasks
- Financial mismanagement
- Less interested in friends, family, and hobbies
- Impaired judgment
- Impulsive (inappropriate behavior, perhaps sexual, towards strangers, perhaps even break the law)

- Loss of empathy & sympathy for others
- Overeating (sugary foods)
- Planning problems
- Paranoia

It might take three years to reach stage three, and two years to work through the severe and critical levels. There are more symptoms each stage, and by now, the disease is winning. Whatever resemblance of the person before the diagnosis fades in painful steps that now include paranoia.

When severe bvFTD grows to critical, a person requires help to eat, walk, bathe, and use the bathroom. At this stage, a bvFTD patient depends on others for daily survival.

Stage 4: Critical bvFTD

It takes an average of five years from diagnosis to stage four bvFTD. Somebody with bvFTD lives an average of 10.5 years from the first symptom manifestation, less than 7.5 after diagnosis.

Somebody with stage four bvFTD requires 24/7 care and is bedridden. Stage four patients require help with all daily tasks. Some symptoms towards the end:

- Abulia
- Acute memory problems
- Difficulty chewing food
- Disinhibition
- Dysphagia (swallowing difficulties)
- Severe apathy
- Speech disability

A *PubMed* study described the final stage. The researchers found 16% fed through tubes, and 46% suffered comorbid somatic diseases[145]. For bvFTD patients, the study concluded:

> *Cardiovascular disease and respiratory disease, mostly pneumonia, were the most frequent causes of death.*

Towards the end, bvFTD patients pool food in their mouth, which causes choking or coughing, causing aspiration pneumonia.

During stage four, people suffer urinary and bowel incontinence. The issue causes acute urinary tract infections and causes sepsis infection throughout the body.

Because of the inactivity, patients often die from blood clots, pulmonary embolism (PE), or deep vein thrombosis (DVT).

Because of the impulsiveness and judgment impairment caused by bvFTD, risk factors for accidental death are much higher than for other dementias. The neurological disorder poses a particular risk in stages one and two when they remain independent and are still driving and living life as usual.

Most Probable Stage 4 Deaths

- Cardiovascular disease
- Respiratory disease (including pneumonia)

Stages Section Sources: American Academy of Neurology[146], Penn Frontotemporal Degeneration Center[147], PubMed Study[148], Hospice of the Valley Dementia Team[149], *Oxford Academic*[150], *Neurology* Study[151], *Science Direct*[152], *JAMA Neurology*[153], *Partners in FTD Care*[154], 2nd *Neurology* Study[155], *Journal of Alzheimer's Disease*[156], 2nd *PubMed* Study[157], Journal of Geriatric Psychiatry and Neurology[158]

Chapter 13: PROGRESSIVE SUPRANUCLEAR PALSY (PSP) STAGES

From the first symptoms, somebody with progressive supranuclear palsy (PSP) lives an average of 6-7 years[159]. The chapter divides the stages as follows:

1. Early-stage
2. Mid-stage
3. Advanced stage
4. Final Act

Early Stage Progressive Supranuclear Palsy (PSP)

Progressive supranuclear palsy (PSP) begins with a jolt. Something unexplainable is wrong. It likely began with neck stiffness. But, we all get stiff, so nobody paid the problem much attention. Nobody had a reason to believe the stiffness is out of the ordinary.

However, the stiffness grows worse and does not go away as normal. Walking becomes more difficult. Movement slows. The loved one, and perhaps others, realize something is amiss, but still perhaps not over-concerned.

The symptoms grow worse, and the loved one suffers the first dizzy spell of many to come. The dizziness grows worse, and at some point, the loved one faints.

If the loved one has not gone to the doctor by now, they do so either from fear or injury from the fainting and consequential fall. PSP patients often fall backward.

Early Stage PSP Symptoms

- Apathy
- Balance issues
- Blurred or double vision
- Eye problems including looking up and down
- Falling backward
- Fatigue
- Irritability
- Mood swings
- Muscle stiffness, often in the neck
- Photophobia (bright lights sensibility)
- Poor judgment
- Reckless behavior

If the loved one had not gone to the doctor by now, they do

so either from fear or injury from the fainting and consequential fall.

At this point, we hope the family doctor refers loved one to a neurologist who recognizes the symptoms, runs the correct tests to narrow the possibilities, and reaches a quick, correct PSP diagnosis.

The diagnosis shocks the patient and loved ones. However, early stages represent the last best time to enjoy the quality time left, but also to put one's final business in order.

There is much important business in this period, including a Living Will, Right of Attorney, financial considerations, neurologist appointments, therapy appointments, and dozens of other important matters one must address while possible.

The activity frenzy helps avoid the emotional issues the diagnosis causes but allows no time to address the shock. Make an appointment with an emotional therapist trained for such neurological disorders. One can extend the quality time left if they overcome depression, anxiety, and other emotions accompanying a fatal, incurable, progressive, debilitating dementia.

Mid Stage Progressive Supranuclear Palsy (PSP)

The patient and loved ones spent much of stage one addressing these types of issues. All while the symptoms pile up and grow worse.

Although the mildest stage of any dementia, I hesitate to say easiest. Stage one is the best life is going to be in the sense of the disorder, but the initial shock and PSP related business make early-stage anything but easy.

When the patient reaches the mid-stage, loved ones likely are just getting their feet under them, but mid-stage brings a new set of problems. Stage one problems worsen.

Joints ache. The tightness in the neck grows more painful, shooting down the back. Headaches grow more frequent and intense.

Mid-Stage Progressive Supranuclear Palsy (PSP) Symptoms

- Balance problems grow more pronounced
- Blepharospasm
- Eye muscle control deteriorates
- Headaches
- Joint pain
- Memory loss
- Mobility problems worsen (might require a wheelchair)
- Neck and back pain
- Sleep problems worsen
- Speech problems (slurred, slow, muffled)

Keeping one's balance proves ever more challenging. The

inability to control eye muscles makes moving dangerous, reading difficult or impossible, increasing falling risk (usually backward). Reduced blinking ability causes dry eyes. PSP produces another mid-stage problem called blepharospasm, a disorder causing involuntary eye closing (lasting a few seconds to several hours).

The mobility problems of stage one turn more severe, and the consequences more brutal. Walking proves difficult, if not impossible, and a wheelchair might already be necessary.

Cognitive issues such as memory and executive skills loss occur in mid-stage. Sleep problems develop or grow worse in mid-stage.

Speech grows more slurred, slow, and muffled. PSP often causes dysphagia (swallowing problems) in mid-stage.

Final Stage Progressive Supranuclear Palsy (PSP)

The shock of early-stage PSP gave way to mid-stage challenges, which gives way to the brutality of late-stage, which gives way to the finality of the final stage.

All symptoms from mid-stage degenerate further. Mid-stage is the stretch everybody has dreaded. However, once the clock starts, reaching this point five or six years from the first symptoms is inevitable for most suffering PSP.

A shell of the person the loved ones once knew now suffers a fate no good person would wish on their worst enemies.

All previous symptoms exacerbate and snowball into a human wrecking ball. Bedridden or in a wheelchair, the PSP overwhelms the loved one.

PSP Final Stage Symptoms

- Bowel dysfunction
- Bladder decline
- Chest infections
- Constipation
- Dementia-related cognitive decline
- Further speaking decline
- Incontinence
- Throat muscles dysfunction (severe swallowing issues)

Previous sleep disruption grows more problematic, in part because of the frequent need to urinate.

A curious PSP combination is one must urinate more often, but urinating itself proves more difficult. Both bowel and bladder problems are prominent in late-stage, often leading to incontinence towards the end.

In the final stage, throat muscle malfunction renders eating impossible, necessitating a feeding tube. Associated problems often cause chest infections.

Verbally communicating continues deteriorating, if not already destroyed, in part because the mouth muscles decline.

While PSP causes cognitive problems, they are not as severe as Alzheimer's and some other dementias. However, in the final stage, PSP causes memory, concentration, and motor skill problems. In most cases, these issues are not severe enough to destroy one's sense of self.

The PSP final stage renders a person near helpless, unable to walk, eat, drink, go to the bathroom, or much of anything at this point. The loved one is in a tough spot, and it only gets worse.

The Final Act

No matter what warning, humans refuse to accept the finality of a loved one's death. In the case of a loved one with progressive supranuclear palsy (PSP), in most cases, we have six or seven years to prepare.

The PSP patient fights through years from diagnosis to reach the final stage. Now the patient struggles through their last stretch in life. For most, the final stretch lasts six to eight weeks[160]. The rapid decline is obvious to those who have followed the patient day to day or week to week.

PSP in the final weeks devastates the patient. A person might slip in and out of consciousness. They are near helpless. Unable to articulate their thoughts, wheelchair, and bed-bound, a person suffers great physical and emotional pain, anxiety, depression, and frustration during this period.

As the clock ticks, the loved one drifts in and out of consciousness.

In their final stretch, the loved one long passed the point where they can take care of basic daily tasks, much less making critical decisions.

Final-stage is the time for the Power of Attorney to kick in and to honor the loved ones previous-stated wishes. These are tough decisions, especially concerning matters where the loved one never expressed their wishes when capable. However, loving somebody means we step up to the plate and prove our love by honoring wishes and making difficult decisions. The designated person likely has been administering such decisions for some time, but now reaches the most difficult one, when to stop treatment.

Once to the final stretch, Hospice typically is called in to help monitor the patient, provide comfort, and monitor medication. Once Hospice comes aboard, the end is near.

PSP patients usually suffer great weight loss down the stretch. Food going down the wrong pipe often causes chest infections.

PSP Cause of Death

Pneumonia, pulmonary embolism, and injuries from falls often cause death[161].

When the time comes, loved ones experience mixed emotions. In part, they feel relief. The loved one no longer suffers. On the other, a person they love no longer graces the living. PSP is a long and winding road that climbs and curves, but there is no mountain top at the end of the road, just a sour, bitter, heart-wrenching ending.

Celebrate Their Life

Losing a loved one under any circumstances crushes the soul, but we must lift ourselves back up and carry on. We must celebrate all the reasons we loved the person and cherish the sweeter memories.

Live on and prosper, as they would wish. Allow time to form scars where the fresh wounds to the soul now torment.

PSP Stages Sources: National Institute of Neurological Disorders and Stroke[162], *eMedicine Health*[163], John Hopkins Medicine[164], *British Medical Journal*[165], European Parkinson's Disease Association EPDA[166], Brain Foundation[167], UCSF[168], Baylor College of Medicine[169], Cleveland Clinic[170], Pacific Movement Disorders Center[171]

V. FTD-RELATED DEMENTIAS RISK FACTORS

We explore behavioral variant frontotemporal dementia (bvFTD) stages in this section.

Science's knowledge of bvFTD leaves much to be desired regarding testing, vaccine, cure, and information such as risk factors.

Chapter 14: BEHAVIORAL VARIANT FRONTOTEMPORAL DEMENTIA (bvFTD) CAUSES & RISK FACTORS

Pinpointing the causes for most dementias, including frontotemporal confounds science. Researchers know genetics cause a third of frontotemporal dementia.

For years, since including Frontotemporal in one of my dementia books, I have called on the government to fund frontotemporal dementia better. We need more research in three areas: causes, accurate and inexpensive tests, and a cure.

While researchers are making progress, they are trudging along because most dementia research money goes to Alzheimer's, Vascular dementia, and Lewy body dementia. I am not suggesting the top three dementias receive too much funding—they do not get enough research money either. But, they get far more than frontotemporal dementia.

Science tells us genetics causes a third of frontotemporal dementia cases, but we know too little concerning the other two-thirds.

bvFTD Behavioral Variant Dementia Risk Factors

We need bigger, better, and long-term studies to root out the causes and risk factors for frontotemporal dementia.

Genetics account for a third, and studies point towards a few culprits for the remaining risk factors.

In a more recent study released in *Tidsskriftet*, researchers reviewed studies in the Cochrane, *Embase*, *PsychInfo*, and PubMed databases.

"The literature suggests associations between diabetes," said study lead author Hege Rasmussen, "head injury and autoimmune disease, and frontotemporal dementia."

Others find enough evidence to list the following as increasing bvFTD risks.

bvFTD Risk Factors

- Diabetes
- Genetics
- Head injuries
- Thyroid disease

Before we move on, let's discuss each potential risk factor.

Diabetes

Researchers link diabetes to several dementias, including frontotemporal.

Angel Golimstok, MD, Department of Neurology at Hospital Italiano and team reviewed 150,000 people in Buenos Aires, Argentina described their findings.

"Previous prospective, large, population-based cohort studies," said Golimstok, "have found that diabetes is associated with an increased risk of cognitive decline and dementia[172]."

The studies in question found diabetes caused a 50-100% risk in the broad category of dementia but provided no specific risks for dementias other than Alzheimer's and vascular.

Dr. Golimstok explained frontotemporal clinical diagnosis studies confirm a higher incidence of type-2 diabetes history. "This is a very significant finding in our population whereas in Latin America," said Golimstok, "diabetes is a highly prevalent disease in over 45 years, with higher percentages of cases than the rest of the world."

Other studies in the United States and around the world drew similar conclusions.

A six-year Swedish study followed a group of seniors age 80-93 and concluded type-2 diabetes, "is associated with accelerated cognitive decline in old age that may result in dementia[173]."

A group of Stanford scientists reviewed several studies focused on a population growing older and type-2 diabetes and higher dementia risk.

The risk for cognitive impairment and dementia increases among those with type 2 diabetes, and insulin resistance represents a potential mechanism by which both Alzheimer's and vascular disease develop.

"Type 2 diabetes is amenable to intervention, and promising therapeutic interventions are under investigation," said lead author Brenna Cholerton, "The abilities to establish risk among specific populations, identify and perhaps prevent progression of the disease early in its process, and institute targeted interventions help to establish type 2 diabetes as an ideal candidate for a precision health approach in dementia[174]."

Type-2 diabetes is almost 100% avoidable or curable through diet, exercise, and other positive health changes. Reduce the risk of frontotemporal dementia and other diseases by preventing or defeating type-2 diabetes.

Genetics

Genetics causes about 10% of frontotemporal dementia (FTD) cases[175].

There is a 50% chance a person with the mutated gene passes it to their child.

Four primary genes related to bvFTD

- C9orf72 (often referred to as the chromosome 9 gene)
- Microtubule-associated protein tau (MAPT, often referred to as "tau")
- Progranulin (GRN or PGRN)
- Valosin-Containing Protein (VCP)

Since there is no bvFTD cure, most physicians do not recommend genetic testing for those who might be at risk.

Head injuries

Traumatic brain injuries increase the risk of frontotemporal dementia (FTD).

A Department of Neurology, Baylor College of Medicine study claims this is because traumatic brain injuries increase microglial levels in the central nervous system[176].

Another study released in Neuroscience concurred with previous studies claiming traumatic brain injuries increases FTD risks[177].

Avoid head injuries!

JERRY BELLER HEALTH RESEARCH INSTITUTE

Thyroid disease

A PubMed review of several studies found a 2.5% FTD risk for those suffering thyroid disease[178].

Another retrospective case-control study in the Journal of Neurology, Neurosurgery, & Psychiatry also drew the same conclusion[179].

They have done far more studies establishing thyroid risk to other dementias, but current data suggest an FTD connection, too.

Chapter 15: PROGRESSIVE SUPRANUCLEAR PALSY RISK FACTORS

According to the Mayo Clinic, science only verifies age as a progressive supranuclear palsy (PSP) risk factor[180]. However, a study released in *Science Direct* found a positive link between high blood pressure and PSP[181]. And PSP attacks men in greater numbers than women.

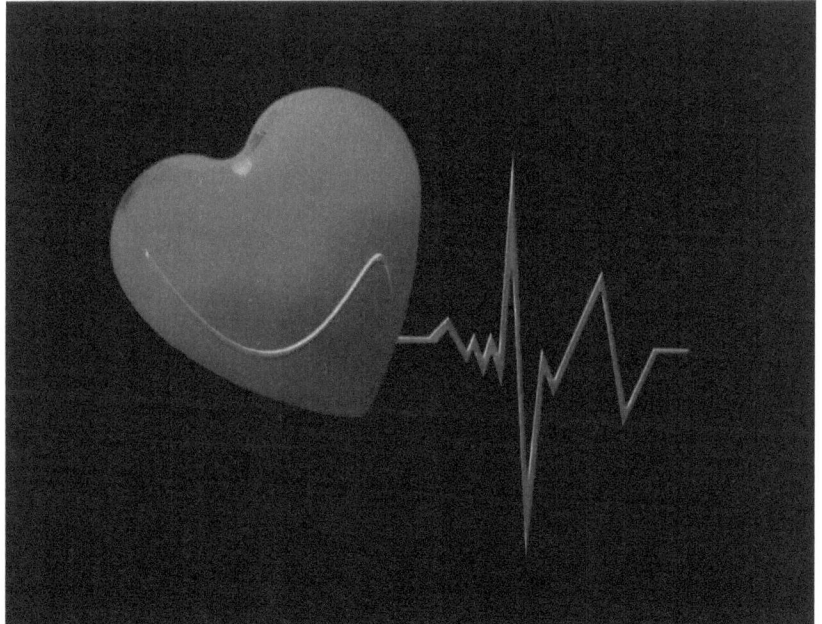

PSP strikes most people when they are sixty or older and is almost nonexistent under forty.

If we build a profile of this killer, progressive supranuclear palsy (PSP) likes victims on the other side of sixty, males somewhat more than women, perhaps with high blood pressure.

It doesn't give us much, and it cannot be the entire picture, meaning we need extensive PSP research. What we do not know outweighs our current knowledge.

JERRY BELLER HEALTH RESEARCH INSTITUTE

VI. BONUS SECTION

Whether diagnosed with dementia or preparing for a rainy day, there are basics everybody should consider.

This section focuses on steps dementia patients (all adults) should address, including forming a care team and understanding various therapy.

While written for dementia patients, I recommend every adult fulfill these tasks before you turn thirty. Waiting is our enemy for these two duties. Be prepared!

The section includes:

1. A starter to-do list for any adult diagnosed with a fatal disease such as dementia.
2. A care team plan.

Chapter 16: Starter To-do List for Somebody and Family once Diagnosed with Dementia.

Dementia patients, loved ones, and family must address several matters early in the disease, including care, financial decisions, living quarters, Living Will, and Power of Attorney.

While you have full or most of your cognitive skills, take care of the listed priorities before diagnosis or when diagnosed. Please do not consider the items covered in this section a complete care list, but a start you tailor to your needs.

Fail to cross these items off the list while you maintain your facilities causes much regret for patients and loved ones.

Your life is your ship, and for now, you remain the captain. Plan how your ship faces the coming storm and, when you can no longer captain the ship yourself, have it already determined who takes over the helm.

Now remains your last best chance to have a substantial say in your future.

Care

Family, loved ones, and dementia patients must make difficult decisions concerning if somebody can become the primary volunteer caregiver. While dementia patients do not require 24/7 care in the early stage, it becomes necessary in the middle to late stages.

Nobody can get through dementia without others providing years of caregiving. While rare dementias kill in months, most dementia patients live for 5-20 years, with dementia growing progressively worse.

Diagnosed with dementia or in perfect health, we all must ask ourselves who would take care of us if dementia or another devastating disorder struck, requiring long-term caregiving.

Most families cannot afford professional caregiving, and the government will not help until towards the end, so family and loved ones must.

In an ideal world, we ask ourselves these tough questions and have a plan in place should something happen. This benefits not only those diagnosed with dementia but also the heroic voluntary caregivers who will see them to the end.

Financial Decisions

There are significant financial decisions to make, and earlier, the better.

Find out how much your insurance covers and the amount you must pay. A kinder world would not burden dementia patients, nor their loved ones, with overwhelming medical care costs.

In the United States and most countries in the world, the majority of dementia costs fall on families.

How Much Does Dementia Cost the Average Family?

With no urine or blood test for most dementia types, neurologists must rely on imaging and other expensive tests, often not to diagnose dementia but to rule out other neurological disorders.

Under the best scenario, related tests, doctor visits saddle the average patient with tens of thousands of dollars in deductibles by the time the neurological team diagnoses them with dementia. For some, such as dementia with Lewy bodies, it might run much higher as it can take up to eighteen months or longer before doctors make a correct diagnosis.

Our health system tells the average person: "Sorry, you have dementia. Oh, by the way, there's the bill."

Doctors, medical professionals, hospitals, drug companies, and others involved in treating dementia must make a living. Even when we factor out overcharging and profiteering, treating dementia would remain expensive.

The average American family's health insurance has deteriorated for years, the premiums growing too high, the deductibles unaffordable, and too many not worth the paper its written, much less the monthly premiums.

Authorities estimate the average cost per dementia patient is $341,840, with families expected to cover 70 percent.

Such a disease becomes a hardship for not only the patient but also their family. The demands, financial and otherwise, on voluntary caregivers often is devastating. Make difficult financial decisions early.

Financial costs vary from one dementia to another and the treatment plan.

Living Quarters

While most dementia patients maintain independence in stage one, at some point, they require help with daily tasks. Will somebody move in with her or him? Does the patient move in with somebody else? Will it become necessary for him or her to move into an assisted living community in later stages? If so, what type?

The person diagnosed should gather loved ones and decide such matters in the beginning. Like somebody on a small island with a hurricane approaching, one must be diligent. While no man or woman can withstand such a storm, they still take precautions to protect themselves and their families.

In part because of financial considerations, most families care for the loved one in the home until symptoms grow critical. Whether a dementia patient ends up in a special need living facility is not a matter of if, but at what point for those who have access.

No matter how much love, care, and attention a voluntary caregiver or loved ones provide a dementia patient, they are ill-equipped to provide for somebody in the disorder's final stretch.

Families without access do the best they can to provide comfort for the loved one but make no mistake, the patient and family benefit if a special needs facility takes over at some point.

Which type of facility depends on which dementia and symptoms. Some dementias cause more cognitive problems, while others greater affect motor skills, some visual, and a few dementias cause more language problems. In the end, many dementias are more alike than not, as the damage to the brain spreads to other areas. Still, depending on the symptoms, different care facilities might be better than others.

Ask your neurologist or local dementia organizations about local facilities trained for your particular type. Hopefully, you live at home and maintain a normal or semi-normal life for years, but have a facility selected when the end grows near.

Living Will

Not to be confused with a Last Will and Testament that distributes assets, a living will focus on medical decisions. NOLO defines a living will.

> *A living will – sometimes called a health care declaration -- is a document in which you describe the kind of health care you want to receive if you are incapacitated and cannot speak for yourself. It is often paired with a power of attorney for health care, in which you name an agent to make health care decisions on your behalf. Some states combine these two documents into one document called an 'advanced directive.'*

It is crucial to document the dementia patient's wishes while you maintain facilities to make such decisions.

Use the Living Will to direct physicians to follow your wishes on what care you receive now and, in the future when you might not maintain your cognitive skills.

Specify end-of-life medical treatment.

NOLO recommends prioritizing life-prolonging medical care, food, and water if you become unconscious, and palliative care, which we soon address[182].

Distribute copies of your living will to loved ones, doctors, insurance providers, and all health care facilities.

Power of Attorney

The American Bar Association describes a power of attorney:

A power of attorney gives one or more persons the power to act on your behalf as your agent. The power may be limited to a particular activity, such as closing the sale of your home or be general in its application. The power may give temporary or permanent authority to act on your behalf. The power may take effect immediately, or only upon the occurrence of a future event, usually a determination that you are unable to act for yourself due to mental or physical disability. The latter is called a "springing" power of attorney. A power of attorney may be revoked, but most states require written notice of revocation to the person named to act for you[183].

It is important to establish a medical power of attorney to empower a trusted loved one to make medical decisions when a patient becomes incapable. If you do not choose the right person, you can almost count on the wrong people making important decisions down the road.

If you're in early stages dementia and reading this, you likely can still think clearly, but this changes as the symptoms worsen. The only way to protect a dementia patient's wishes when they lose their cognitive decision making is by naming a power of attorney in advance.

Once you name a power of attorney, cover some dos and don'ts. After all, you are trusting another person with your life. Like with your doctors, speak your mind while you can and let people know what you expect.

As NOLO pointed out, some states merge the living will and power of attorney into an advanced directive. Whether together or separate, I recommend all adults, and particularly those diagnosed with dementia draw up a medical living will and name a power of attorney.

The starter to-do list provides a starting point for dementia patients, families, and any adult.

Once diagnosed, both the person diagnosed and loved ones must unite and build your to-do list. Add whatever makes sense for you and your unique situation.

Let's next cover a few key members of a dementia care team.

Chapter 17: CARE TEAM

The National Institute on Aging recommends building a care team.

The team includes an art therapist, mental health counselor, occupational therapist, palliative care specialist, physical therapist, and a speech therapist[184].

Art therapist

The art therapist reduces stress by engaging the patient in music and other expressive arts.

Since dementia causes enormous anxiety and mood swings, art therapists use music and art to soothe patients and assist caregivers. Most everybody responds to music. Some pump our blood and makes us want to shake our bodies to the rhythm. Other music helps us focus and achieve maximum concentration.

Some music geared towards dementia patients relaxes and calms. Music is a godsend!

Art is not a task but a love affair. Some say within each of us is an artist starving to escape. Art therapists use music and art as a brilliant tool to treat dementia anxiety, attention decline, sleep problems, etc.

Mental health counselors

A neurological disorder, dementia attacks the brain and inhibits cognitive skills. Mental health counselors help patients and families plan for the future and cope with the shock, hurt, and pain resulting from the diagnosis.

Most individuals and families suffer chronic mental stress when doctors diagnose a member with dementia.

Find a mental health counselor trained in dementia.

Turn to their expertise and do not allow the neurological disorder to destroy the remaining quality of life for the patient, or respond as a family in a way where dementia destroys many lives by one sweeping event.

Occupational therapists

The occupational therapist helps patients bathe, dress, eat, and perform daily tasks.

We think of the routine daily tasks as second nature, and it is as long as the neurons, pathways, arteries, heart, and brain perform as normal. When suffering a stroke or neurological disorder like dementia, we quickly learn nothing is second nature anymore. Like a child, dementia patients often must relearn how to perform basic tasks.

Occupational therapists help patients remain independent and then semi-independent, as long as possible, extending the quality of life. An occupational therapist is instrumental in treating most dementias.

Palliative care specialist

The palliative care specialist minimizes symptoms from diagnosis to the end. You or a loved one need somebody who addresses symptoms as soon as they arise, so find a quality palliative care specialist.

They extend the quality of life and reduce suffering.

Physical therapists

Physical therapists help motors skills by leading patients through exercise.

Although dementia is known as a mental disorder, what affects the brain affects the body and vice versa. Find a physical therapist trained to work with your specific dementia.

If you've seen somebody suffering Parkinsonism or other neurological disorders affecting movement, you have an idea of the problems some dementias cause, even in the earliest stages.

A physical therapist helps maintain balance and strength, allowing a person to walk and move on their own. As dementia progresses, so does the physical therapist's importance.

Speech therapists

The speech therapist addresses speech and swallowing problems, issues present in early dementia symptoms for some types, and eventually becomes a problem for most dementias.

What is the value of verbalizing one's thoughts, understanding what a loved one says, and swallowing our food without choking or causing infection by sending it down the wrong pipe?

These are issues speech therapists excel. The ones I've observed are passionate about helping people retrain the mind to overcome aphasia and swallowing problems.

Find a speech (and other types of) therapist trained in treating your specific type of dementia. These different listed therapists can minimize the long nightmare following a dementia diagnosis.

Chapter 18: LETTER TO CONGRESS

DEAR U.S. CONGRESS, NATIONS OF THE WORLD, & WEALTHY HUMANS

We call on the United States and the governments of the world to spend less on war and walls and more on Alzheimer's and dementia research.

If aliens were attacking us from another planet, I presume the nations of the world would unite against a common enemy. That is what I propose now.

The enemy I refer to does not come from another planet but threatens humans no less. Alzheimer's and dementia strike an American every 68 seconds and somebody worldwide every 30 seconds.

The nations of the world can save millions of lives and billions of dollars.

We need necessary funding to:

1. Discover the exact cause (s) of Alzheimer's and other dementias.
2. Develop accurate testing for Alzheimer's and other dementias.
3. Develop a vaccine to wipe out Alzheimer's and other dementias like we did polio.

Alzheimer's and dementia grow at a rate that will destroy the economies of most countries if we do not become more proactive.

We can save trillions of dollars for future generations if we invest now in discovering the exact cause (s), a vaccine to prevent it from happening, and other steps to defeat this horrifying disease.

Alzheimer's and other dementias threaten every family in all nations.

We can do little for those with late-stage dementia, but the proposed steps might save millions of lives and trillions of dollars by diagnosing the different dementias early and treating them before they do significant damage.

Beller Health calls on politicians, corporations, and wealthy individuals to step forward to help win the war against dementia.

CONCLUSION

Thank you for reading this book. We covered a good amount of material.

Dementia is a cruel neurological disorder that robs people of their personalities, executive skills, memories, talents, language, voice, motor capabilities, and all that makes us individual humans.

Alzheimer's and Dementia

Although Alzheimer's disease (AD) is the most prevalent, we learned AD is to dementia what China is to Asia. Alzheimer's represents 60-80% of dementia, but 19 dementia types account for 99 percent.

Dementia Spares No Demographic

Dementia's reputation is known as an old folk's disease but strikes people all ages. Most dementia is not genetic, although certain types such as Huntington's disease are 100% familial.

Most Dementia is Incurable

Most dementia is incurable, but—if caught early enough—neurosurgeons can treat and sometimes reverse normal pressure hydrocephalus.

Dementia Prevalence

The first section focused on dementia as a general category. We learned 850,000 people in the UK have dementia, compared to 5.8 Americans and 50 million people worldwide.

Dementia Categories

We divided the 19 dementias into six categories:

- Lewy Body/Parkinsonism related dementias
- Alzheimer's related dementias
- Frontotemporal lobar degeneration related dementias
- Primary progressive aphasia related dementias
- Vascular dementias
- Other dementias

19 Dementia Types

Lewy Body/Parkinsonism Related Dementias

1. *Dementia with Lewy Bodies*
2. *Parkinson's Disease Dementia*
3. Corticobasal Syndrome

Alzheimer's Related Dementias

4. Typical Alzheimer's Disease
5. *Posterior Cortical Atrophy*
6. *Down Syndrome with Alzheimer's*
7. *Limbic-predominant Age-related TDP-43 Encephalopathy (LATE)*
8. Early-onset Alzheimer's

Frontotemporal Lobar Degeneration Related Dementias

9. *Behavioral Variant Frontotemporal Dementia*
10. Progressive Supranuclear Palsy

Primary Progressive Aphasia Related Dementias

11. *Nonfluent Primary Progressive Aphasia (nfvPPA)*

12. Logopenic Progressive Aphasia (LPA)

Vascular Dementia

13. *Cortical Vascular Dementia*
14. *Binswanger Disease*

Other Dementias

15. *Normal Pressure Hydrocephalus*
16. *Huntington's Disease*
17. *Korsakoff Syndrome*
18. *Creutzfeldt-Jakob Disease*
19. Amyotrophic Lateral Sclerosis

We examined frontotemporal related dementias, defining and exploring causes, prevalence, symptoms, and stages.

THE END

Of

FRONTOTEMPORAL RELATED DEMENTIAS

THANK YOU FOR READING

Thank you for reading the entire book. While this is not a literary work to enjoy, I hope you gained useful knowledge of posterior cortical atrophy.

If you benefitted from this book, please take a moment to share your thoughts in a review. Reader reviews help other readers make educated decisions about this book before purchasing.

Book Review link for Frontotemporal Related Dementias

or

https://www.amazon.com/dp//B07XTJGYB4

Look for annual updates to my health books, as I follow new studies and add any helpful information I find. Health and fitness are top priorities, and the heart and brain are my specialties.

I hope you develop the habits suggested in this book. Good luck on your health journey. Live long and prosper, my friend.

All the best,
Jerry Beller & Beller Health

BELLER HEALTH BOOKS

Beller Health Research Institute specializes in the heart and brain, and published the following Jerry Beller book series:

- Arrhythmia Series
- Vascular Disease Series
- 2020 Dementia Overview Series
- 19 Dementia Types Series

Please continue to view the books in each series.

Dementia Types, Symptoms, Stages, & Risk Factors Series

This book series is the first to cover each of the 19 primary dementia types.

2020 Dementia Overview Series

Whereas in the *Dementia Types, Symptoms, Stages, and Risk Factors* series, each book covers a different dementia type, this series focuses on groups of dementias.

1. Dementia Types, Symptoms, & Stages
2. *Lewy Body/Parkinsonism Dementias*
3. *Vascular Dementia*
4. *Frontotemporal Dementia (FTD)*
5. Alzheimer's Related Dementias
6. *Prevent or Slow Dementia*

Other Beller Health Books

You can view or purchase all Beller Health Books on Amazon at the following web address:

https://amzn.to/2TpDr8e

ABOUT THE AUTHOR

Jerry Beller is the lead author and researcher at Beller Medical Research Institute. Beller distinguished himself three times in the medical world by being the first to write and publish books on particular dementia fields.

He wrote the first book covering all 15 primary dementia types, which he since expanded to cover nineteen. Beller followed this accomplishment by writing a book on each dementia type. He broke medical ground a third time when he published the first book on the new dementia category LATE.

When the world struggled to grasp the difference between Alzheimer's disease and China, Beller explained:

Alzheimer's is only one dementia, much like China is only one country in Asia. Just as we do not want to ignore the other countries in Asia because China is the largest, nor do we want to ignore the less prevalent dementia types.

Despite his accomplishments, he remains humble. "Until we win the dementia war, I've no reason to celebrate," Beller said. "If we win the war during my lifetime, I will celebrate with a few hundred brothers and sisters around the world who share my passion. Until then, we have too much work left to worry about accolades and legacies."

When not researching dementia, Jerry enjoys life with his wife of thirty-plus years, Nicola, and their two children.

Visit Jerry Beller:

https://bellerhealth.com

1 'What Is Dementia?', Alzheimer's Disease and Dementia <https://alz.org/alzheimers-dementia/what-is-dementia> [accessed 18 September 2019].

2 'What Is Dementia? Symptoms, Types, and Diagnosis', National Institute on Aging <https://www.nia.nih.gov/health/what-dementia-symptoms-types-and-diagnosis> [accessed 18 September 2019].

3 'What Is Dementia?', *Alzheimer's Society* <https://www.alzheimers.org.uk/about-dementia/types-dementia/what-dementia> [accessed 18 September 2019].

4 'Dementia' <https://www.who.int/news-room/fact-sheets/detail/dementia> [accessed 18 September 2019].

5 'Risk Factors' <https://stanfordhealthcare.org/medical-conditions/brain-and-nerves/dementia/risk-factors.html> [accessed 20 September 2019].

6 W. M. van der Flier and P. Scheltens, 'Epidemiology and Risk Factors of Dementia', *Journal of Neurology, Neurosurgery & Psychiatry*, 76.suppl 5 (2005), v2–7 <https://doi.org/10.1136/jnnp.2005.082867>.

7 Kent Allen, 'Dementia Rates to Grow for African Americans, Hispanics', *AARP* <http://www.aarp.org/health/dementia/info-2018/dementia-alzheimer-cases-grow-nonwhites.html> [accessed 20 September 2019].

8 Elizabeth Rose Mayeda and others, 'Inequalities in Dementia Incidence between Six Racial and Ethnic Groups over 14 Years', *Alzheimer's & Dementia: The Journal of the Alzheimer's Association*, 12.3 (2016), 216–24 <https://doi.org/10.1016/j.jalz.2015.12.007>.

9 'African Americans at Higher Dementia Risk than Other Racial Groups', *Reuters*, 10 March 2016 <https://www.reuters.com/article/us-health-dementia-race-u-s-idUSKCN0WC2X5> [accessed 20 September 2019].

10 Steve Ford, 'Likelihood of Dementia "Higher among Black Ethnic Groups"', *Nursing Times*, 2018 <https://www.nursingtimes.net/news/research-and-innovation/likelihood-of-dementia-higher-among-black-ethnic-groups-08-08-2018/> [accessed 21 September 2019].

11 'Dementia' <https://www.who.int/news-room/fact-sheets/detail/dementia> [accessed 21 September 2019].

[12] 'Women and Alzheimer's', *Alzheimer's Disease and Dementia* <https://alz.org/alzheimers-dementia/what-is-alzheimers/women-and-alzheimer-s> [accessed 21 September 2019].

[13] 'Dementia Facts', *Dementia Consortium* <https://www.dementiaconsortium.org/dementia-facts/> [accessed 21 September 2019].

[14] 'Dementia' <https://www.who.int/news-room/fact-sheets/detail/dementia> [accessed 21 September 2019].

[15] 'Why Is Dementia Different for Women?', *Alzheimer's Society* <https://www.alzheimers.org.uk/blog/why-dementia-different-women> [accessed 21 September 2019].

[16] Jessica L. Podcasy and C. Neill Epperson, 'Considering Sex and Gender in Alzheimer Disease and Other Dementias', *Dialogues in Clinical Neuroscience*, 18.4 (2016), 437–46 <https://www.ncbi.nlm.nih.gov/pmc/articles/PMC5286729/> [accessed 21 September 2019].

[17] 'WHO | Life Expectancy', *WHO* <http://www.who.int/gho/mortality_burden_disease/life_tables/situation_trends_text/en/> [accessed 21 September 2019].

[18] 'Products - Data Briefs - Number 328 - November 2018', 2019 <https://www.cdc.gov/nchs/products/databriefs/db328.htm> [accessed 21 September 2019].

[19] Jacqui Thornton, 'WHO Report Shows That Women Outlive Men Worldwide', *BMJ*, 365 (2019), l1631 <https://doi.org/10.1136/bmj.l1631>.

[20] 'Why Do Women Live Longer Than Men?', *Time* <https://time.com/5538099/why-do-women-live-longer-than-men/> [accessed 21 September 2019].

[21] 'Dementia' <https://www.who.int/news-room/fact-sheets/detail/dementia> [accessed 20 September 2019].

[22] 'Alzheimer's Disease: Facts & Figures', *BrightFocus Foundation*, 2015 <https://www.brightfocus.org/alzheimers/article/alzheimers-disease-facts-figures> [accessed 4 September 2019].

[23] 'Facts for the Media', *Alzheimer's Society* <https://www.alzheimers.org.uk/about-us/news-and-media/facts-media> [accessed 20 September 2019].

[24] 'Countries With The Highest Rates Of Deaths From Dementia',

WorldAtlas <https://www.worldatlas.com/articles/countries-with-the-highest-rates-of-deaths-from-dementia.html> [accessed 20 September 2019].

[25] 'World Alzheimer Report 2018 - The State of the Art of Dementia Research: New Frontiers', *NEW FRONTIERS*, 48.

[26] 'ALZHEIMERS/DEMENTIA DEATH RATE BY COUNTRY', *World Life Expectancy* <https://www.worldlifeexpectancy.com/cause-of-death/alzheimers-dementia/by-country/> [accessed 24 September 2019].

[27] 'Alzheimer Europe - Research - European Collaboration on Dementia - Cost of Dementia - Regional/National Cost of Illness Estimates' <https://www.alzheimer-europe.org/Research/European-Collaboration-on-Dementia/Cost-of-dementia/Regional-National-cost-of-illness-estimates> [accessed 26 September 2019].

[28] 'Publications | NATSEM' <https://www.natsem.canberra.edu.au/publications/?publication=economic-cost-of-dementia-in-australia-2016-2056> [accessed 22 September 2019].

[29] 'Dementia UK Report', *Alzheimer's Society* <https://www.alzheimers.org.uk/about-us/policy-and-influencing/dementia-uk-report> [accessed 22 September 2019].

[30] 'Dementia Statistics – U.S. & Worldwide Stats', *BrainTest*, 2015 <https://braintest.com/dementia-stats-u-s-worldwide/> [accessed 23 September 2019].

[31] 'Newsroom | Northwestern Mutual - 2018 C.A.R.E. Study', *Newsroom | Northwestern Mutual* <https://news.northwesternmutual.com/2018-care-study> [accessed 22 September 2019].

[32] 'ALZHEIMERS/DEMENTIA DEATH RATE BY COUNTRY'.

[33] 'Alzheimer Europe - Research - European Collaboration on Dementia - Cost of Dementia - Regional/National Cost of Illness Estimates'.

[34] 'Publications | NATSEM'.

[35] 'Dementia UK Report'.

[36] 'Dementia Statistics – U.S. & Worldwide Stats'.

[37] NeuRA, 'Frontotemporal Dementia', *NeuRA*, 2016 <https://www.neura.edu.au/health/frontotemporal-dementia/> [accessed 15 January 2019].

[38] 'Frontotemporal Dementia', *Memory and Aging Center*

<https://memory.ucsf.edu/dementia/ftd> [accessed 28 October 2019].

[39] 'What Are Frontotemporal Disorders?', *National Institute on Aging* <https://www.nia.nih.gov/health/what-are-frontotemporal-disorders> [accessed 28 October 2019].

[40] Daniela Galimberti and Elio Scarpini, 'Genetics of Frontotemporal Lobar Degeneration', *Frontiers in Neurology*, 3 (2012) <https://doi.org/10.3389/fneur.2012.00052>.

[41] T. B. Gislason and others, 'The Prevalence of Frontal Variant Frontotemporal Dementia and the Frontal Lobe Syndrome in a Population Based Sample of 85 Year Olds', *Journal of Neurology, Neurosurgery & Psychiatry*, 74.7 (2003), 867–71 <https://doi.org/10.1136/jnnp.74.7.867>.

[42] 'Disease Overview', *Association for Frontotemporal Degeneration* <https://www.theaftd.org/understandingftd/ftd-overview> [accessed 18 February 2018].

[43] 'Fast-Facts-Final-11-12.Pdf' <https://www.theaftd.org/wp-content/uploads/2009/05/Fast-Facts-Final-11-12.pdf> [accessed 18 February 2018].

[44] 'Frontotemporal Dementia' <https://www.hopkinsmedicine.org/health/conditions-and-diseases/dementia/frontotemporal-dementia> [accessed 30 October 2019].

[45] 'FAQs', *AFTD* <https://www.theaftd.org/what-is-ftd/faqs/> [accessed 30 October 2019].

[46] 'Frontotemporal Dementia - Health Encyclopedia - University of Rochester Medical Center' <https://www.urmc.rochester.edu/encyclopedia/content.aspx?contenttypeid=134&contentid=77> [accessed 30 October 2019].

[47] NeuRA.

[48] NeuRA.

[49] Allan Ajifo, *English: Caricature on the Differences between Right and Left Brain Sides.*, 2014, https://www.flickr.com/photos/125992663@N02/14414603887/ <https://commons.wikimedia.org/wiki/File:Right_brain.jpg> [accessed 18 February 2018].

[50] 'Disease Overview'.

[51] 'Fast-Facts-Final-11-12.Pdf'.

[52] NeuRA.

[53] 'The Penn FTD Center | Behavioral Variant Frontotemporal Dementia (BvFTD)' <https://ftd.med.upenn.edu/about-ftd-related-disorders/what-are-these-conditions/behavioral-variant-frontotemporal-dementia-bvftd> [accessed 14 January 2019].

[54] 'Behavioral Variant Frontotemporal Dementia', *Memory and Aging Center* <https://memory.ucsf.edu/behavioral-variant-frontotemporal-dementia> [accessed 14 January 2019].

[55] Michelle Leahy, 'Fast Facts about Frontotemporal Degeneration', 1.

[56] 'Frontotemporal Dementia' <https://stanfordhealthcare.org/medical-conditions/brain-and-nerves/dementia/types/frontotemporal-dementia.html> [accessed 5 December 2019].

[57] Christer Nilsson and others, 'Age-Related Incidence and Family History in Frontotemporal Dementia: Data from the Swedish Dementia Registry', *PLoS ONE*, 9.4 (2014) <https://doi.org/10.1371/journal.pone.0094901>.

[58] Galimberti and Scarpini.

[59] Gislason and others.

[60] 'Progressive Supranuclear Palsy', *Nhs.Uk*, 2017 <https://www.nhs.uk/conditions/progressive-supranuclear-palsy-psp/> [accessed 5 December 2019].

[61] 'Progressive Supranuclear Palsy Fact Sheet | National Institute of Neurological Disorders and Stroke' <https://www.ninds.nih.gov/disorders/patient-caregiver-education/fact-sheets/progressive-supranuclear-palsy-fact-sheet> [accessed 4 December 2019].

[62] 'Progressive Supranuclear Palsy (PSP) | Asceneuron' <https://www.asceneuron.com/progressive-supranuclear-palsy-psp> [accessed 5 December 2019].

[63] 'Parkinson-Plus Syndromes. Clues to Diagnosis, Multiple System Atrophy, Progressive Supranuclear Palsy', 2019 <https://emedicine.medscape.com/article/1154074-overview#a3> [accessed 5 December 2019].

[64] 'Progressive Supranuclear Palsy Fact Sheet | National Institute of Neurological Disorders and Stroke'.

[65] R. W. Shin and others, 'Hydrated Autoclave Pretreatment Enhances Tau Immunoreactivity in Formalin-Fixed Normal and Alzheimer's Disease Brain Tissues', *Laboratory Investigation; a Journal of Technical Methods and Pathology*, 64.5 (1991), 693–702.

[66] Nicolas Sergeant, André Delacourte, and Luc Buée, 'Tau Protein as a Differential Biomarker of Tauopathies', *Biochimica et Biophysica Acta (BBA) - Molecular Basis of Disease*, The Biology and Pathobiology of Tau, 1739.2 (2005), 179–97 <https://doi.org/10.1016/j.bbadis.2004.06.020>.

[67] 'Progressive Supranuclear Palsy (PSP) | Asceneuron'.

[68] 'Behavioral Variant Frontotemporal Dementia | Memory and Aging Center' <https://memory.ucsf.edu/behavioral-variant-frontotemporal-dementia> [accessed 18 February 2018].

[69] '7 Stages of Frontotemporal Dementia | Exploring Dementia, One Stage at a Time' <http://exp.stagesofdementia.net/7-stages-of-frontotemporal-dementia/> [accessed 18 February 2018].

[70] 'Frontotemporal Dementia' <http://alzheimer.ca/en/Home/About-dementia/Dementias/Frontotemporal-Dementia-and-Pick-s-disease> [accessed 18 February 2018].

[71] 'Pick Disease of the Brain: Causes, Symptoms, and Diagnosis' <https://www.healthline.com/health/picks-disease> [accessed 18 February 2018].

[72] 'Primary Progressive Aphasia - an Overview | ScienceDirect Topics' <https://www.sciencedirect.com/topics/medicine-and-dentistry/primary-progressive-aphasia> [accessed 18 February 2018].

[73] 'Diseases That Cause Dementia | Dementia Care Notes', *Dementia Care Notes, India*, 2010 <https://dementiacarenotes.in/dementia/causes-of-dementia/> [accessed 18 February 2018].

[74] 'Frontotemporal Dementia', 2017 <https://www.centogene.com/science-education/centopedia/factsheets/ngs-panel-genetic-testing-for-frontotemporal-dementia.html> [accessed 18 February 2018].

[75] 'Dementia Symptoms and Diagnosis - Illnesseses and Conditions | NHS Inform' <https://www.nhsinform.scot/illnesses-and-conditions/brain-nerves-and-spinal-cord/dementia/dementia-symptoms-

and-diagnosis/dementia-symptoms-and-diagnosis> [accessed 18 February 2018].

[76] 'Frontotemporal Dementia: A Brain Disease That Challenges Definitions of Mental Illness: Page 5 of 5 | Psychiatric Times' <http://www.psychiatrictimes.com/dementia/frontotemporal-dementia-brain-disease-challenges-definitions-mental-illness/page/0/4> [accessed 18 February 2018].

[77] Virginia E. Sturm and others, 'Prosocial Deficits in Behavioral Variant Frontotemporal Dementia Relate to Reward Network Atrophy', *Brain and Behavior*, 7.10 (2017) <https://doi.org/10.1002/brb3.807>.

[78] Joyce Fraker and others, 'The Role of the Occupational Therapist in the Management of Neuropsychiatric Symptoms of Dementia in Clinical Settings', *Occupational Therapy In Health Care*, 28.1 (2014), 4–20 <https://doi.org/10.3109/07380577.2013.867468>.

[79] 'Frontotemporal Dementia: Symptoms And Treatment Explained After 40-Year-Old Dies From Disease' <http://www.huffingtonpost.co.uk/entry/frontotemporal-dementia-symptoms-and-treatment-explained_uk_58e21d77e4b0c777f7889878> [accessed 18 February 2018].

[80] 'Frontotemporal Dementia' <http://alzheimer.ca/en/Home/About-dementia/Dementias/Frontotemporal-Dementia-and-Pick-s-disease> [accessed 18 February 2018].

[81] 'Frontotemporal Dementia | Memory and Aging Center' <https://memory.ucsf.edu/frontotemporal-dementia> [accessed 18 February 2018].

[82] 'The Effect of Changed Behaviors of Frontotemporal Dementia on the Stress Level of Informal Caregivers - ProQuest' <https://search.proquest.com/openview/5c9cf3e4aeb9a2bd0689d8de20c82729/1?pq-origsite=gscholar&cbl=18750&diss=y> [accessed 18 February 2018].

[83] Mette Sagbakken and others, 'Dignity in People with Frontotemporal Dementia and Similar Disorders — a Qualitative Study of the Perspective of Family Caregivers', *BMC Health Services Research*, 17 (2017) <https://doi.org/10.1186/s12913-017-2378-x>.

[84] 'PinFTDcare_Newsletter_Spring_2017.Pdf' <https://www.theaftd.org/wp-content/uploads/2017/04/PinFTDcare_Newsletter_Spring_2017.pdf> [accessed 18 February 2018].

[85] 'Frontotemporal Dementia - an Overview | ScienceDirect Topics' <https://www.sciencedirect.com/topics/neuroscience/frontotemporal-dementia> [accessed 18 February 2018].

[86] 'Symptoms', *Nhs.Uk* <https://www.nhs.uk/conditions/frontotemporal-dementia/symptoms/> [accessed 18 February 2018].

[87] 'What Is Pick's Disease, What Are the Symptoms of Frontotemporal Dementia and What Is a Sufferer's Life Expectancy?', *The Sun*, 2017 <https://www.thesun.co.uk/living/2907739/picks-disease-symptoms-frontotemporal-dementia/> [accessed 18 February 2018].

[88] 'Dementia', *American Speech-Language-Hearing Association* <https://www.asha.org/public/speech/disorders/dementia/> [accessed 18 February 2018].

[89] 'Frontotemporal Dementia: Types, Symptoms, Treatment' <https://www.medicalnewstoday.com/articles/316113.php> [accessed 18 February 2018].

[90] 'Frontotemporal (Frontal Lobe) Dementia: Causes, Symptoms, and Treatments' <https://www.webmd.com/alzheimers/guide/frontotemporal-dementia#1> [accessed 18 February 2018].

[91] 'Inflammatory Pathways Link to Obsessive Behaviors in Frontotemporal Dementia - Neuroscience News' <http://neurosciencenews.com/obsessive-behavior-ftd-6490/> [accessed 18 February 2018].

[92] 'Frontotemporal Disorders: Hope Through Research | National Institute of Neurological Disorders and Stroke' <https://www.ninds.nih.gov/Disorders/Patient-Caregiver-Education/Hope-Through-Research/Frontotemporal-Disorders> [accessed 18 February 2018].

[93] 'Frontotemporal Dementia | Johns Hopkins Medicine Health Library' <https://www.hopkinsmedicine.org/healthlibrary/conditions/nervous_system_disorders/frontotemporal_dementia_134,77> [accessed 18 February 2018].

[94] 'Posterior Cortical Atrophy', *Wikipedia*, 2018 <https://en.wikipedia.org/w/index.php?title=Posterior_cortical_atrophy&oldid=858211681> [accessed 12 January 2019].

[95] 'Behavioral Variant Frontotemporal Dementia | Memory and Aging Center'.

[96] 'Frontotemporal Disorders: Hope Through Research | National Institute of Neurological Disorders and Stroke'.

[97] 'Frontotemporal Dementia | Johns Hopkins Medicine Health Library'.

[98] 'Symptoms'.

[99] 'Frontotemporal Dementia'.

[100] 'Dementia Symptoms and Diagnosis - Illnesseses and Conditions | NHS Inform'.

[101] Sagbakken and others.

[102] 'Frontotemporal Dementia | Memory and Aging Center'.

[103] 'Frontotemporal (Frontal Lobe) Dementia: Causes, Symptoms, and Treatments'.

[104] 'The Effect of Changed Behaviors of Frontotemporal Dementia on the Stress Level of Informal Caregivers - ProQuest'.

[105] 'Frontotemporal Dementia: A Brain Disease That Challenges Definitions of Mental Illness: Page 5 of 5 | Psychiatric Times'.

[106] Sturm and others.

[107] 'Inflammatory Pathways Link to Obsessive Behaviors in Frontotemporal Dementia - Neuroscience News'.

[108] Fraker and others.

[109] 'Frontotemporal Dementia - an Overview | ScienceDirect Topics'.

[110] 'Frontotemporal Disorders: Hope Through Research | National Institute of Neurological Disorders and Stroke' <https://www.ninds.nih.gov/Disorders/Patient-Caregiver-Education/Hope-Through-Research/Frontotemporal-Disorders>

[accessed 18 February 2018].

111 'Frontotemporal Dementia: Types, Symptoms, Treatment'.

112 '7 Stages of Frontotemporal Dementia | Exploring Dementia, One Stage at a Time'.

113 'Frontotemporal Dementia'.

114 'Frontotemporal Dementia: Symptoms And Treatment Explained After 40-Year-Old Dies From Disease'.

115 'Pick Disease of the Brain: Causes, Symptoms, and Diagnosis'.

116 'Primary Progressive Aphasia - an Overview | ScienceDirect Topics'.

117 'PinFTDcare_Newsletter_Spring_2017.Pdf'.

118 'What Is Pick's Disease, What Are the Symptoms of Frontotemporal Dementia and What Is a Sufferer's Life Expectancy?'

119 'Dementia'.

120 'Diseases That Cause Dementia | Dementia Care Notes'.

121 'Frontotemporal Dementia'.

122 'Behavioral Variant Frontotemporal Dementia | Memory and Aging Center'.

123 '7 Stages of Frontotemporal Dementia | Exploring Dementia, One Stage at a Time'.

124 'Frontotemporal Dementia'.

125 'Pick Disease of the Brain: Causes, Symptoms, and Diagnosis'.

126 'Primary Progressive Aphasia - an Overview | ScienceDirect Topics'.

127 'Diseases That Cause Dementia | Dementia Care Notes'.

128 'Frontotemporal Dementia'.

129 'Dementia Symptoms and Diagnosis - Illnesseses and

Conditions | NHS Inform'.

[130] 'Frontotemporal Dementia: A Brain Disease That Challenges Definitions of Mental Illness: Page 5 of 5 | Psychiatric Times'.

[131] Sturm and others.

[132] Fraker and others.

[133] 'Frontotemporal Dementia: Symptoms And Treatment Explained After 40-Year-Old Dies From Disease'.

[134] 'Frontotemporal Dementia'.

[135] 'Frontotemporal Dementia | Memory and Aging Center'.

[136] 'The Effect of Changed Behaviors of Frontotemporal Dementia on the Stress Level of Informal Caregivers - ProQuest'.

[137] Sagbakken and others.

[138] 'PinFTDcare_Newsletter_Spring_2017.Pdf'.

[139] 'Frontotemporal Dementia - an Overview | ScienceDirect Topics'.

[140] 'Frontotemporal Disorders: Hope Through Research | National Institute of Neurological Disorders and Stroke'.

[141] 'Frontotemporal Dementia | Johns Hopkins Medicine Health Library'.

[142] 'Progressive Supranuclear Palsy - Symptoms', *Nhs.Uk*, 2018 <https://www.nhs.uk/conditions/progressive-supranuclear-palsy-psp/symptoms/> [accessed 7 December 2019].

[143] 'Progressive Supranuclear Palsy Fact Sheet | National Institute of Neurological Disorders and Stroke' <https://www.ninds.nih.gov/disorders/patient-caregiver-education/fact-sheets/progressive-supranuclear-palsy-fact-sheet> [accessed 7 December 2019].

[144] William W. Seeley and others, 'Frontal Paralimbic Network Atrophy in Very Mild Behavioral Variant Frontotemporal Dementia', *Archives of Neurology*, 65.2 (2008), 249–55 <https://doi.org/10.1001/archneurol.2007.38>.

[145] Norman Sartorious, 'Comorbidity of Mental and Physical Diseases: A Main Challenge for Medicine of the 21st Century', *Shanghai Archives of Psychiatry*, 25.2 (2013)

<https://doi.org/10.3969/j.issn.1002-0829.2013.02.002>.

[146] Ian T.S. Coyle-Gilchrist and others, 'Prevalence, Characteristics, and Survival of Frontotemporal Lobar Degeneration Syndromes', *Neurology*, 86.18 (2016), 1736–43 <https://doi.org/10.1212/WNL.0000000000002638>.

[147] 'The Penn FTD Center | Advanced Illness and Long-Term Care' <https://ftd.med.upenn.edu/living-with-ftd-related-disorders/long-term-care> [accessed 21 January 2019].

[148] J. Diehl-Schmid and others, 'Behavioral Variant Frontotemporal Dementia: Advanced Disease Stages and Death. A Step to Palliative Care', *International Journal of Geriatric Psychiatry*, 32.8 (2017), 876–81 <https://doi.org/10.1002/gps.4540>.

[149] 'Hospice-and-FTD_Hospice-of-the-Valley-2011-Ppt-Online-Version.Pdf' <https://www.theaftd.org/wp-content/uploads/2011/10/Hospice-and-FTD_Hospice-of-the-Valley-2011-ppt-online-version.pdf> [accessed 21 January 2019].

[150] Muireann Irish and others, 'Differential Impairment of Source Memory in Progressive Versus Non-Progressive Behavioral Variant Frontotemporal Dementia', *Archives of Clinical Neuropsychology*, 27.3 (2012), 338–47 <https://doi.org/10.1093/arclin/acs033>.

[151] E. Mioshi and others, 'Clinical Staging and Disease Progression in Frontotemporal Dementia', *Neurology*, 74.20 (2010), 1591–97 <https://doi.org/10.1212/WNL.0b013e3181e04070>.

[152] Marshal F. Folstein, Susan E. Folstein, and Paul R. McHugh, '"Mini-Mental State": A Practical Method for Grading the Cognitive State of Patients for the Clinician', *Journal of Psychiatric Research*, 12.3 (1975), 189–98 <https://doi.org/10.1016/0022-3956(75)90026-6>.

[153] William W. Seeley and others, 'Frontal Paralimbic Network Atrophy in Very Mild Behavioral Variant Frontotemporal Dementia', *Archives of Neurology*, 65.2 (2008), 249–55 <https://doi.org/10.1001/archneurol.2007.38>.

[154] 'January-2014.Pdf' <https://www.theaftd.org/wp-content/uploads/2011/09/January-2014.pdf> [accessed 21 January 2019].

[155] Petra Steinacker and others, 'Serum Neurofilament Light Chain

in Behavioral Variant Frontotemporal Dementia', *Neurology*, 91.15 (2018), e1390–1401 <https://doi.org/10.1212/WNL.0000000000006318>.

156 Rebekah M. Ahmed and others, 'Characterizing Sexual Behavior in Frontotemporal Dementia', ed. by Marc Sollberger, *Journal of Alzheimer's Disease*, 46.3 (2015), 677–86 <https://doi.org/10.3233/JAD-150034>.

157 Tiffany W. Chow and others, 'Trajectories of Behavioral Disturbance in Dementia', *Journal of Alzheimer's Disease : JAD*, 31.1 (2012), 143–49 <https://doi.org/10.3233/JAD-2012-111916>.

158 Sarah J. Banks and Sandra Weintraub, 'Neuropsychiatric Symptoms in Behavioral Variant Frontotemporal Dementia and Primary Progressive Aphasia', *Journal of Geriatric Psychiatry and Neurology*, 21.2 (2008), 133–41 <https://doi.org/10.1177/0891988708316856>.

159 'What Is the Prognosis of Progressive Supranuclear Palsy (PSP)?' <https://www.medscape.com/answers/1154074-99795/what-is-the-prognosis-of-progressive-supranuclear-palsy-psp> [accessed 12 December 2019].

160 'Four Stages of PSP (PSP Association, UK)', *Brain Support Network*, 2013 <https://www.brainsupportnetwork.org/four-stages-of-psp-psp-association-uk/> [accessed 12 December 2019].

161 'What Is the Prognosis of Progressive Supranuclear Palsy (PSP)?'

162 'Progressive Supranuclear Palsy Fact Sheet | National Institute of Neurological Disorders and Stroke' <https://www.ninds.nih.gov/Disorders/Patient-Caregiver-Education/Fact-Sheets/Progressive-Supranuclear-Palsy-Fact-Sheet> [accessed 12 December 2019].

163 'Progressive Supranuclear Palsy Life Expectancy & PSP Treatment', *EMedicineHealth* <https://www.emedicinehealth.com/progressive_supranuclear_palsy/articl e_em.htm> [accessed 12 December 2019].

164 'Progressive Supranuclear Palsy' <https://www.hopkinsmedicine.org/health/conditions-and-diseases/progressive-supranuclear-palsy> [accessed 12 December 2019].

165 Huw R. Morris, Nicholas W. Wood, and Andrew J. Lees, 'Progressive Supranuclear Palsy (Steele-Richardson-Olszewski Disease)', *Postgraduate Medical Journal*, 75.888 (1999), 579–84

<https://doi.org/10.1136/pgmj.75.888.579>.

166 European Parkinson's Disease Association, 'Progressive Supranuclear Palsy: Myths, Misconceptions and Facts about PSP' <https://www.epda.eu.com/latest/news/progressive-supranuclear-palsy-myths-misconceptions-and-facts-about-psp/> [accessed 12 December 2019].

167 'Progressive Supranuclear Palsy Life Expectancy & PSP Treatment'.

168 'Progressive Supranuclear Palsy', *Memory and Aging Center* <https://memory.ucsf.edu/dementia/progressive-supranuclear-palsy> [accessed 12 December 2019].

169 'Progressive Supranuclear Palsy (PSP)', *Baylor College of Medicine* <https://www.bcm.edu/healthcare/care-centers/parkinsons/conditions/progressive-supranuclear-palsy> [accessed 12 December 2019].

170 'Progressive Supranuclear Palsy (PSP Disease)', *Cleveland Clinic* <https://my.clevelandclinic.org/health/articles/6096-progressive-supranuclear-palsy> [accessed 12 December 2019].

171 'Progressive Supranuclear Palsy Symptoms & Treatment', *Pacific Movement Disorders* <https://www.pacificneuroscienceinstitute.org/movement-disorders/conditions/atypical-parkinsonism/progressive-supranuclear-palsy/> [accessed 12 December 2019].

172 Angel Golimstok and others, 'Cardiovascular Risk Factors and Frontotemporal Dementia: A Case–Control Study', *Translational Neurodegeneration*, 3 (2014), 13 <https://doi.org/10.1186/2047-9158-3-13>.

173 Linda B. Hassing and others, 'Type 2 Diabetes Mellitus Contributes to Cognitive Decline in Old Age: A Longitudinal Population-Based Study', *Journal of the International Neuropsychological Society: JINS*, 10.4 (2004), 599–607 <https://doi.org/10.1017/S1355617704104165>.

174 Brenna Cholerton and others, 'Type 2 Diabetes, Cognition, and Dementia in Older Adults: Toward a Precision Health Approach', *Diabetes Spectrum : A Publication of the American Diabetes Association*, 29.4 (2016), 210–19

<https://doi.org/10.2337/ds16-0041>.

¹⁷⁵ Lisa Kinsley and HyungSub Shim, 'FTD/PPA Family Caregiver and Professional Education and Support Conference 2012', 2012, 9.

¹⁷⁶ Ali Jawaid and others, 'Traumatic Brain Injury May Increase the Risk for Frontotemporal Dementia through Reduced Progranulin', *Neuro-Degenerative Diseases*, 6.5–6 (2010), 219–20 <https://doi.org/10.1159/000258704>.

¹⁷⁷ '(PDF) Traumatic Brain Injury Causes Frontotemporal Dementia and TDP-43 Proteolysis', *ResearchGate* <http://dx.doi.org/10.1016/j.neuroscience.2015.05.013>.

¹⁷⁸ Natalie D Weder and others, 'Frontotemporal Dementias: A Review', *Annals of General Psychiatry*, 6 (2007), 15 <https://doi.org/10.1186/1744-859X-6-15>.

¹⁷⁹ Weder and others.

¹⁸⁰ 'Progressive Supranuclear Palsy Symptoms & Treatment'.

¹⁸¹ Soniya V. Rabadia and others, 'Hypertension and Progressive Supranuclear Palsy', *Parkinsonism & Related Disorders*, 66 (2019), 166–70 <https://doi.org/10.1016/j.parkreldis.2019.07.036>.

¹⁸² Betsy Simmons Hannibal and Attorney, 'How to Write a Living Will', *Www.Nolo.Com* <https://www.nolo.com/legal-encyclopedia/how-write-living-will.html> [accessed 21 November 2019].

¹⁸³ 'Power of Attorney' <https://www.americanbar.org/groups/real_property_trust_estate/resources/estate_planning/power_of_attorney/> [accessed 22 November 2019].

¹⁸⁴ 'Treatment and Management of Lewy Body Dementia', *National Institute on Aging* <https://www.nia.nih.gov/health/treatment-and-management-lewy-body-dementia> [accessed 24 April 2019].

www.ingramcontent.com/pod-product-compliance
Lightning Source LLC
Chambersburg PA
CBHW030648220526
45463CB00005B/1684